THE DOCTOR'S KIDNEY DIETS

A NUTRITIONAL GUIDE TO

MANAGING AND SLOWING

THE PROGRESSION OF

CHRONIC KIDNEY DISEASE

MANDIP S. KANG, MD, FASN

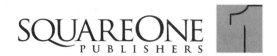

SQUAREONE
PUBLISHERS

The information and advice contained in this book are based upon the research and the personal and professional experiences of the author. They are not intended as a substitute for consulting with a healthcare professional. The publisher and author are not responsible for any adverse effects or consequences resulting from the use of any of the suggestions or procedures discussed in this book. All matters pertaining to your physical health should be supervised by a healthcare professional. It is a sign of wisdom, not cowardice, to seek a second or third opinion.

COVER DESIGNER: Jeannie Tudor
RECIPE ILLUSTRATIONS: Vicki Chelf
TYPESETTER: Gary A. Rosenberg
IN-HOUSE EDITOR: Joanne Abrams

Square One Publishers
115 Herricks Road
Garden City Park, NY 11040
(516) 535-2010 • (877) 900-BOOK
www.squareonepublishers.com

Library of Congress Cataloging-in-Publication Data
Kang, Mandip S.
  The doctor's kidney diets : a nutritional guide to managing and slowing the progression of chronic kidney disease / Mandip S. Kang, MD, FASN.
    pages cm
  Includes
bibliographical references and index.
  ISBN 978-0-7570-0373-8 (pbk.)
  1.
Kidneys—Diseases. 2. Kidneys—Diseases—Nutritional aspects. 3. Kidneys—Diseases—Diet therapy. 4. Self-care, Health. I. Title.
  RC903.K36
2015
  616.6'10654—dc23
                    2015018370

Printed in the United States of America

10   9   8   7   6   5   4   3   2   1

Contents

*I dedicate this book to those who have a passion
for helping others in the face of adversity.
Your kindness and courage to step forward
truly sets you apart from the rest of us.*

Acknowledgments

I am indebted to Rudy Shur, Publisher; Joanne Abrams, Executive Editor; and other members of the talented Square One Publishers staff whose skilled hands made this book a reality. Your patience, support, and belief in my message were enormously helpful. Sincere thanks also go to Barbara Albers Hill, whose gift for creating reader-friendly text will allow this book to benefit kidney patients everywhere.

Thank you to Uhling Consulting's registered dietitians: Aubrey Uhling, RD, CDE; Christina Caple, RD; and Meghan Smith, RD, for helping to create new recipes and evaluate dietary information. Appreciation also goes to Jacquelyn Beyrami, MS, RD, CSR; Nancee Vanderpluym, MS, RD; and Kara Abbas, MS, RD, CSR, for their input and analysis of many of the recipes.

I am thankful for great minds that taught me the art and science of kidney diseases at Wake Forest University School of Medicine, especially John Burkart, MD, who trained me during my fellowship and was kind enough to review this book. Many thanks to my former colleagues at the University of Utah School of Medicine's Nephrology Department. Special thanks also go to my colleagues at the Southwest Kidney Institute, who inspire and motivate me daily, and to my patients, whose many stories taught me that making small changes can indeed make a big difference in one's health.

Finally, a heartfelt thank-you to my wonderful family: to my loving wife, Manjit Kang, RN, for assisting with recipes and helping review the book through professional eyes; to my insightful daughter, Amrita, for her proofreading skills; and to my son, Aneel, for his invaluable computer assistance, research expertise, and unconditional support. Lastly, thank you to my brother for his gifts of confidence and encouragement. My family's love and generosity are truly the foundation of this book.

Foreword

In 1953, Homer Smith, one of the "fathers" of nephrology (the study of kidney disease), suggested that the kidney may have played an important role in the evolution of many biological species, including mankind. Along the course of these evolutionary processes, the kidney became responsible for many processes needed to maintain health. These processes go way beyond the obvious one of removing excess fluids from the body—in other words, urine production. It is what is not so obvious—the toxins, chemicals, salt and other minerals that are in that urine—that make the kidney the important and complex organ that it is. Our kidneys work twenty-four hours a day, seven days a week to prevent these chemicals and minerals from accumulating so we can remain healthy. When our kidneys are diseased, our health is threatened. One of the major sources of the chemicals and minerals that may accumulate is dietary intake. It is not surprising, then, that dietary choices are an important part of routine health maintenance, a significant step in minimizing strain on the kidneys, and a vital part of the overall treatment for patients with chronic kidney illness or kidney failure treated with dialysis.

The Doctor's Kidney Diets by Mandip Kang, MD, FASN, is an invaluable guide to the dietary management and treatment of kidney disease. It is exactly what both the patient and the doctor needed.

Dietary management of kidney disease does not have to be hard. In fact, with the recipes included in this book, it can even be enjoyable. Dr. Kang has combined his years of knowledge treating patients with kidney disease and other illnesses with his passion for patient care. The book is very informative and easy to read. He recognizes that there is more than "one" kidney diet, and that we need to individualize therapy to get it right. The goal is to make the dietary part of the treatment for a patient with kidney disease—usually, a lifelong condition—manageable, meaningful, and effective. In following this aspect of treatment, the reader should feel better and enjoy a more active, longer, and more satisfying life. I believe this book outlines a great way to do just that. It is my hope that you enjoy the book, the recipes, and most of all, greater health.

John Burkart, MD
Professor of Nephrology/Medicine
Wake Forest University Medical Center
Winston Salem, North Carolina

He that takes medicine and neglects diet,
wastes the skills of the physician.

Chinese Proverb

$\mathcal{I}$ntroduction

In the United States today, it has been estimated that 26 million adults have chronic kidney disease, and millions of others are at increased risk due to rising rates of the two most common causes of CKD—hypertension (high blood pressure) and diabetes. It is not surprising, then, that kidney disease has been classified as an epidemic. While people diagnosed with CKD need to know that it is considered a lifelong condition, they also need to know that this disorder is *absolutely manageable*. Underlying causes can be addressed, and a healthier lifestyle can be adopted with an eye toward slowing the progression of the disease. My years as a nephrologist (kidney doctor) have shown me that, whether you're treating CKD alone or juggling the management of several health conditions, diet is a significant part of your treatment plan. By following the diet that meets your needs, you can keep your body's fluid and chemical levels in better balance, improving the chance of stabilizing your kidney function and enhancing your overall health. That is why I wrote *The Doctor's Kidney Diets*—to guide you in understanding and following a kidney-friendly eating plan so that you can enjoy the greatest health possible.

When someone is diagnosed with chronic kidney disease, kidney specialists and nutritionists emphasize the importance of diet to prevent the worsening of the disease, and to avoid the symptoms and complications that can develop due to this lifelong problem. Too often, though, patients find the information given to them inadequate or confusing, especially when several different disorders are involved, each with its own dietary limitations. The purpose of this book is to fill that information gap and empower you to improve your health through the foods you eat and the lifestyle changes you make. The facts and recommendations found in this book have been culled from scientific studies, from the expertise of a panel of nutritionists, and—perhaps most important—from years spent treating thousands of people with kidney disease.

Part One of this book focuses on the kidneys—both their function and their dysfunction—and on the importance of diet in the treatment of CKD. It lays the groundwork of information you need to manage chronic kidney disease.

Chapter 1 reviews the vital tasks performed by the kidneys. This information is important because the goal of CKD treatment includes —although it is not limited to—compensating for the tasks that your kidneys can no longer perform. Understanding kidney function is basic to understanding the management of kidney disease.

Once you've learned about the work performed by the kidneys, you'll be ready to learn what happens when the kidneys are less able to do their job. Chapter 2 focuses on the nature, causes, and stages of chronic kidney disease. It also introduces you to your essential role as a member of your own healthcare team.

In Chapter 3, the spotlight is on nutrition. Which nutrients may have to be limited in your diet, and why? Which foods can cause further kidney damage, and which can actually help you safeguard kidney function? Chapter 3 lays out the facts and also explores important topics such as using vitamin-and-mineral supplements, choosing healthy beverages, dining out, and more.

Many people think that there is only one "renal diet"—one eating plan that is right for everyone with CKD. The truth is that, depending on the stage of CKD, any concurrent medical conditions, and other factors, your doctor may recommend one of several diets, or may combine two or more diets to meet your special needs. Chapter 4 not

2

only explains the diets that are most commonly prescribed for people with CKD, but also provides valuable tips for successfully using each plan to manage your health.

Dietary changes are of crucial importance to everyone with CKD, but beyond diet, there is much you can do to manage your CKD. Chapter 5 focuses on the many healthy lifestyle changes you can make, from getting regular exercise to limiting the use of alcohol and caffeine. Some of these changes may be easy to implement, and some may prove more challenging, but all can make a positive difference in the way you feel on a daily basis as well as in your long-term health.

Although it's important to understand the "why's" of making smart food choices, I know that dietary principles alone won't help you feel better. You need to put those principles into practice by making and enjoying kidney-friendly dishes. That's why Part Two of *The Doctor's Kidney Diets* offers over fifty dietitian-created recipes designed specifically for people with CKD. From breakfasts to desserts, from side dishes to snacks, these dishes are not only easy to follow but also easy to love. Each one starts by listing the specific diets with which it is a good match and ends by listing Nutritional Facts, including calories, protein, carbohydrates, fiber, total fat, saturated fat, trans fat, cholesterol, phosphorus, potassium, and sodium. You'll even find the Diabetic Exchanges per portion. This takes the guesswork out of finding appealing dishes that match your dietary needs and restrictions. Keep in mind, though, that all dietary decisions should be made under the guidance of your healthcare team. I urge you to share these recipes with your doctor and dietitian so that you can determine together how the dishes can be incorporated into your menu plan.

I've tried to make the information in this book easy to understand and to keep my use of medical terminology to a minimum. But some special terms are necessary to explain kidney function, kidney disease, and nutrition. With this in mind, I've created a Glossary (page 171) that explains the terms used in this book as well as the terms you're likely to hear when working with you healthcare team. Turn to it whenever you want to double-check the meaning of a health-related word or phrase.

Throughout this book, I emphasize the importance of under-standing your condition and its treatment. My experience has been that knowledge and active involvement in your healthcare plan are the keys to a good outcome. This book provides a great start, but you'll want to keep adding to your knowledge. That's why I have compiled a comprehensive Resources list (see page 183), which guides you to solid sources of information on kidney-friendly diets, specific foods and nutrients, laboratory tests, and other aspects of CKD treatment, as well as treatment for related conditions such as diabetes and heart disease. The websites and organizations listed in the Resources section can provide you with the information you need to begin the successful management of your condition and to face any new challenges you may encounter along the way.

In my practice, I have seen my patients reap the benefits of dietary and lifestyle changes—as well as patient education regarding the disease process—and these benefits have often been significant. In many individuals, kidney function has stabilized; in others, the time from diagnosis to dialysis has been greatly prolonged. It is my hope that, armed with *The Doctor's Kidney Diets*, you will be able to enhance your long-term health and manage, slow, or even halt the course of chronic kidney disease.

PART ONE

Your Kidneys
and Your Health

If you've been diagnosed with chronic kidney disease (CKD) or have learned that you are at risk of developing this condition, you may feel that you have entered a whole new world. There is suddenly a great deal to learn about why your kidneys aren't working properly; what this means to your overall health; and how you can help guard against a further decline in kidney function. Your doctor will be your first source of information, of course, and you can expect to have many conversations about kidney function, lab test results, related medical conditions, and the significant impact dietary choices can have on your kidneys' health. You may also discuss what you can do to improve your general fitness level. The knowledge you gain during your office visits will be a wonderful start to your understanding of CKD. But you don't want to stop learning the moment you leave your doctor's office, because the more you know about your condition and the importance of kidney-friendly eating, the more you will be able to participate in your own health care and feel truly in control. Part One can be a vital part of this learning process.

Chapter 1 presents important background information about kidney function. You may be surprised by the diverse tasks—from filtering out wastes to safeguarding bones—that healthy kidneys perform to maintain good health. It's crucial to understand this, because one of the purposes of a CKD diet is to help you preserve your health even when your kidneys are unable to do their usual jobs.

Chapter 2 offers clear information about the nature, causes, and progression of chronic kidney disease, which is the focus of this book. It also begins to acquaint you with your role as a member of your healthcare team.

Chapter 3 further explores your need to be actively involved in your own treatment plan by throwing a spotlight on the critical area of nutrition. This information-packed chapter helps you understand the impact that diet has on the kidneys, and focuses on certain important nutrients—protein, potassium, phosphorus, and more—that you may have to monitor during your treatment for CKD. Most important, it shows you how, in conjunction with your healthcare team, you can choose foods that will lessen the strain on your kidneys, help preserve kidney function, and allow you to meet your nutritional needs.

Chapter 4 reviews the diets that are most commonly prescribed for people with CKD, depending on the stage of CKD; whether there are concurrent medical conditions such as diabetes, heart disease, and kidney stones; and other factors. As you will learn, your doctor and nutritionist will help you tailor your diet to your particular needs, which will likely change over time. This chapter will explain the reason for each type of diet and provide valuable tips and guidelines for successfully using each meal plan to manage your health.

By the time you reach Chapter 5, the final section of Part One, you'll know a great deal about treating CKD through the thoughtful selection and preparation of foods. But there are many more steps you can take to improve your health and well-being. This chapter explores the most important of these steps, from working actively and productively with healthcare professionals to getting regular exercise, giving up tobacco, and limiting alcohol use.

You can do so much to feel better and live a longer, more active, more satisfying life. So let's begin the journey to improved health by learning some basics about the kidneys.

1

$\mathcal{U}$nderstanding How Healthy Kidneys Function

Your kidneys are amazing organs that are essential to overall good health. In fact, you may be surprised to learn just how many jobs your kidneys perform to keep your body working properly! As you read the sections that follow, you'll discover what is involved in healthy kidney function and understand the important role your kidneys play in maintaining the well-being of your blood, heart, bones, and more. Armed with this information, you'll gain a new appreciation of the need to protect these hard-working organs.

WHERE YOUR KIDNEYS ARE LOCATED

It makes sense to begin your exploration of kidney function by seeing where these organs are located in the body. Your two kidneys are situated along the muscular wall of your back, on either side of your spine between your rib cage and waist. The right kidney is placed a bit lower than the left to allow room for your liver. Each kidney is bean-shaped and, when healthy, is about the size of your fist.

As you read further, you'll learn that your kidneys oversee the filtering of the blood, which is delivered to each kidney through a special artery. (See Figure 1.1.) As the wastes are filtered out of the blood, the kidneys produce urine, which flows out of the kidneys to the *bladder*—a sort of storage tank—through thin tubes called *ureters*. When your bladder becomes full, a tiny muscle called the *sphincter* can be relaxed to allow the stored urine to exit your body through another tube, the *urethra*. Your kidneys, bladder, and connecting tubes combine to form your *urinary system,* sometimes referred to as the *renal system.* (See Figure 1.2.)

WHAT HEALTHY KIDNEYS DO

Although kidneys average only about five inches in length, they have a lot of job responsibilities. As you're about to see, the daily operation of these organs is pretty complex. This is because most of the tasks that kidneys perform are intertwined with other events that take place in your body. Below, you'll learn the main roles that the kidneys play to maintain health.

Removing Waste Materials, Toxins, and Excess Minerals from Your Body

One important role of the kidneys is to cleanse your blood of unneeded chemicals that can become dangerous if allowed to build up to toxic levels. Some of these waste materials and toxins come from the foods you take in, portions of which your body uses for energy and self-repair. Medications, too, contribute to the buildup of wastes. As the component nutrients and chemicals from these sources are carried around your body, your organs and tissues take what they need and send the excess back to the blood. Additional waste materials get into your bloodstream from the normal break-down of active tissues such as your muscles.

To remove these unwanted, unneeded substances, your kidneys continually filter the blood that passes through them. More than forty gallons of blood are cleansed by healthy kidneys each day—enough to fill the hot water heater in an average home! Here's what happens during the process: Inside each of your kidneys are lots of tiny filter-ing units called *nephrons.* (See Figure 1.1.) Each nephron houses an even smaller *glomerulus*—a network of tiny blood vessels that use

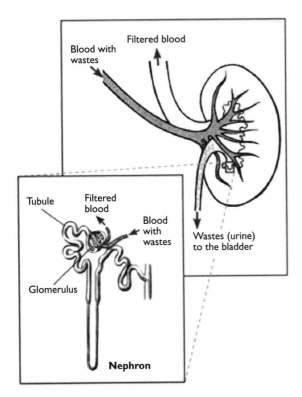

Figure 1.1. How Blood Enters and Leaves the Kidney.
Unfiltered blood is delivered to the kidneys through renal arteries. After wastes are filtered out by the filtering units known as nephrons, the blood is returned to the bloodstream.

Figure 1.2. The Urinary (Renal) System.
This front view of the urinary system shows that your kidneys connect to the bladder via the ureters. Urine produced by your kidneys passes through the ureters, collecting in your bladder for eventual release through the urethra.

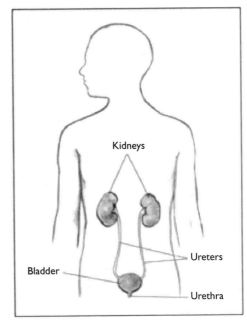

your blood pressure to separate wastes and toxins from the necessary materials in your blood. This filtered waste becomes part of your urine and eventually exits your body through the urinary system shown in Figure 1.2. Meanwhile, the newly cleansed blood goes back to your bloodstream and continues circulating around your body.

As the kidneys filter toxic waste products from the blood, they also remove excess amounts of vital chemicals known as *electrolytes*, which include sodium, calcium, potassium, magnesium, and phosphorus. Although these chemicals are needed for essential functions such as the regulation of heart beat (heart rhythm), if they build up in the blood, the consequences can be serious. Healthy kidneys are able to maintain constant electrolyte levels in the blood.

Balancing Your Body's Fluids

The water that's stored in your body enables your cells, tissues, and organs to work correctly. Therefore, it's important to maintain just the right level of this fluid. Your body is able to remove any unneeded water during the blood filtering process, releasing it into your urine. Or it can hold onto additional fluid if you happen to need it. The task of balancing the water in your body is overseen by your kidneys.

Your blood is composed of 90 percent water, which is what allows it to carry blood cells, nutrients, and other substances around your body. Extra water retained in your body naturally leads to increased blood volume, while a reduced amount of water—say, because of excess sweating or illness—makes your blood volume lower. Both of these conditions can lead to problems if not corrected. To head off trouble, your body releases a hormone called *ADH*, or *antidiuretic hormone*, whenever it senses that your blood volume is low. This hormone tells your kidneys to reduce and concentrate the urine they produce, thereby keeping extra water in your blood. Conversely, if an increase in blood volume is sensed by your body, no ADH is released. This makes your kidneys retain less water and increase their urine output until your blood volume returns to a proper level. When your blood volume drops again, ADH is released once more.

The amount of sodium (salt) in your blood also helps regulate your body's fluid. This may not surprise you, since sodium is closely linked to the retention of water. A drop in your body's sodium level signals a drop in blood volume, and your body responds by sending an enzyme called *renin* into your bloodstream. The renin triggers events that lead your kidneys to hold onto extra sodium and water. On the other hand, when increased sodium is sensed, signaling higher blood volume, your body answers by producing less renin. This tells your kidneys to filter and excrete more sodium and water until your blood levels return to normal. This cycle begins again if your sodium level drops. As you can see, both ADH and renin help to regulate the amount of water in your body, aiming for a fluid balance that contributes to healthy blood pressure, which is further discussed below.

Regulating Your Blood Pressure

Your blood pressure is a measure of the force exerted on your blood vessel walls by circulating blood. This pressure is mainly due to your heart's pumping action, which varies according to the volume of your blood. When there's an increase in your body's fluid level and, in turn, your blood volume, your heart has to pump harder to push blood into already crowded vessels. This creates higher blood pressure, a condition that can lead to serious health problems, including damage to the kidneys' glomeruli and a decreased ability of the kidneys to perform their filtering job.

When your blood pressure goes up, healthy kidneys help reduce it by filtering and excreting extra water and sodium as described in the previous section. The resulting decreased blood volume lowers your blood pressure and lessens the strain on your blood vessels and heart. If your blood pressure drops below a healthy level, signaling low blood volume, you've seen that your kidneys hold onto more sodium and water to correct the situation. Interestingly, the production of renin that triggers this correction also prompts other events that makes your blood vessels contract. This vessel constriction also helps to elevate low blood pressure.

It is clear that your body's water and sodium levels are major contributors to the state of your blood pressure. A change in the level of either substance automatically sets off a series of corrective events, with your kidneys playing a key role in maintaining stability. Amazingly, however, your kidneys do even more.

Maintaining Your Body's Acid-Base Balance

In order to keep all its systems working properly, your body needs to maintain a healthy balance between acids and bases, sometimes called *body pH* or *acid-base homeostasis.* Your body pH can be compared to the pH of a swimming pool, which owners keep within a desired range by adding extra acid or base chemicals whenever necessary. The maintenance of a proper acid-base balance is another job performed by your kidneys.

As your kidneys go about their filtering work, they can sense when acid levels in your blood have moved beyond healthy limits, usually due to illness or consumption of the wrong foods. Since acid levels that are too high or too low can lead to health problems, your kidneys work to balance your pH. This delicate task is largely accomplished by controlling the level of *bicarbonate,* a very strong base found in the body. If extra bicarbonate is needed to offset high acid levels, your kidneys hold onto extra amounts of this base during blood filtration. If too much bicarbonate exists in your body, your kidneys work to restore a healthy pH by straining out more of this chemical and releasing it into your urine. Your kidneys also regulate pH by excreting excess acids, such as uric acid, which the body forms as a by-product of activities such as the metabolism of food. As with other jobs your kidneys do, this process takes place in a cycle, with changes being made as needed to maintain an acid-base balance.

Protecting the Health of Your Bones

Strange as it may sound, your kidneys are also helpful to your bones. If your bones are to remain strong, your blood has to contain the right levels of two important minerals: phosphorus and calcium. Healthy kidneys oversee this mineral balance during the blood filtering process, holding onto the amount that's needed and straining out any excess. However, if your kidneys can't filter out enough phosphorus, a condition usually brought on by illness, this mineral builds up in your blood. Your body then senses that your phosphorus and calcium levels are out of sync and releases a chemical called *PTH*, or *parathyroid hormone*. PTH helps re-balance these levels by making extra calcium move out of your bones and into your bloodstream. Over the long term, this corrective activity can make your bones weak and brittle.

Healthy kidneys also contribute to bone health by helping your body absorb calcium—one of the main building blocks of bones. They do this by turning the vitamin D you obtain from food, supplements, and exposure to the sun into a form your body can use. You see, the vitamin D you take in is biologically inactive and, by itself, isn't helpful to the body. Your kidneys change inactive vitamin D into an active form called *calcitriol*, which helps your intestinal tract absorb the right amount of calcium during digestion. When necessary, calcitriol also works with PTH to help regulate your calcium and phosphorus levels.

Controlling the Production of Red Blood Cells

You've already read that healthy kidneys keep your blood free of unneeded chemicals and water. But did you know that these hard-working organs also regulate the blood by overseeing the creation of new red blood cells?

Your red blood cells are produced in your bone marrow. These important cells are in charge of delivering oxygen from your lungs to your cells and tissues. Red blood cells also carry away carbon dioxide for release from the body as you exhale.

To ensure that your body has the number of red blood cells it needs, healthy kidneys release a hormone called *EPO*, or *erythropoietin*, which stimulates the bone marrow to make more cells. The production of EPO can decrease in the presence of some illnesses, leading to too few red blood cells—a condition commonly known as *anemia*. EPO production can also increase if anemia or high altitude causes a drop in the amount of oxygen in your blood. You see, lower blood oxygen tells your body that more red blood cells are necessary and additional EPO is needed to increase production. Controlling the manufacture of red blood cells—like the other jobs your kidneys perform—is a matter of balance.

IN CONCLUSION

Your kidneys are like powerful machines that operate around the clock. Under the right conditions, this special machinery can work for many, many years without a breakdown. When kidney disease is present, however, these organs become less efficient at performing their important tasks. The jobs of filtering wastes and regulating chemicals are no longer done properly, which upsets the state of balance needed to keep your body's systems working smoothly. Serious health problems can result.

Chapter 2 discusses kidney disease in some depth by looking at its causes, its progression, its diagnosis, and its symptoms. Perhaps most important, it begins exploring the important role you can play in managing your kidney problems and supporting kidney function.

2

$\mathcal{U}$nderstanding Kidney Disease

As you read in Chapter 1, your body exists in a state of balance during times of good health, and your kidneys are responsible for many of the tasks that contribute to this balance. It's easy to see why ongoing problems with kidney function can have a major impact on your overall health. The information presented in this chapter will give you a clear understanding of the nature, common causes, and progression of *chronic kidney disease* (*CKD*), the focus of this book. You will also learn some basics about the goal of CKD treatment. Finally, you will get valuable advice about your own role in helping protect your kidney function.

WHAT IS KIDNEY DISEASE?

Kidney disease, sometimes called *renal disease,* is a general term for any condition or injury that lessens your kidneys' ability to filter waste materials from your blood and perform other necessary functions, such as the regulation of body chemicals and the production of hormones. In some instances, kidney damage can happen quickly, but in the majority of cases, the loss of renal function is more gradual. In fact, you may not even know that you have kidney problems until your organs become quite impaired, because symptoms don't usually surface right away! The following are three main types of kidney disease.

Congenital Kidney Disease

This category accounts for many cases of childhood kidney disease. Congenital disease includes structural problems or blockages that were present at birth, as well as hereditary kidney disorders. These problems often have life-long effects.

Acute Kidney Injury (AKI)

Acute kidney injury (AKI) occurs suddenly due to infection, injury, surgery, the ingestion of poison, or a severe reaction to a medication or the contrast dye used in imaging procedures. The kidney damage that is associated with AKI sometimes improves, but it can also become permanent, leading to chronic kidney disease, which is discussed below.

Chronic Kidney Disease (CKD)

Chronic kidney disease, or *CKD,* is the most prevalent form of kidney disorder by far. At present, 26 million American adults have CKD, and the number of cases is continuing to increase among all age groups. Unlike congenital or acute disease, this disorder usually brings a slow decline in kidney function over months or even years. While the condition is usually symptom-free early on, kidney health can be expected to worsen if corrective steps aren't taken. Fortunately, as you'll learn later in the chapter, there is much you can do to combat this disorder.

WHAT ARE THE COMMON CAUSES OF CHRONIC KIDNEY DISEASE?

As you've just read, kidney problems that occur because of trauma, infection, physical problems, or inherited disorders can sometimes lead to chronic kidney disease. Immune system illnesses such as lupus can also bring about kidney problems, as can recurrent infections, some cancer treatments, and the improper use of pain relievers and some prescription drugs. However, nearly three-quarters of adult CKD cases develop because of three health conditions: diabetes, high blood pressure, and an inflammatory disease known as glomerulonephritis.

Diabetes

Diabetes is the leading cause of kidney disease and end-stage renal disease (ESRD). Over 29 million Americans are diabetic, and the numbers are rising. More than 40 percent of diabetics develop kidney disease.

People with diabetes have higher-than-normal levels of the sugar known as *glucose* in their blood. There are three main types of diabetes. *Gestational diabetes* occurs in expectant women who have no diabetic history, and usually disappears at the pregnancy's end. In *type 1 diabetes,* the blood sugar level is high because the body produces little or no insulin, the hormone that enables body cells to absorb glucose from the blood. In *type 2 diabetes,* the blood sugar level rises even though insulin is present, because the body's cells are unable to use the hormone properly. In all cases, glucose remains in the blood rather than being absorbed and used by the cells.

In both type 1 and type 2 diabetes, over time, the high levels of glucose in the blood damage the filtering units of the kidneys, impairing the organs' ability to remove wastes and water from the blood. The damaged filtering units also cause blood pressure to rise, which, as you'll learn below, can further harm the kidneys.

High Blood Pressure

High blood pressure, also called *hypertension,* is the second leading cause of chronic kidney disease. This condition has been found to account for about 28 percent of all CKD cases.

As discussed in Chapter 1 (see page 11), in high blood pressure, the force of blood against the walls of the blood vessels is greater than normal, making the heart work harder to circulate the blood throughout the body. When pressure remains high over time, the blood vessels—including the large arteries leading to the kidneys and the tiny blood vessels (glomeruli) within the kidneys—begin to stretch to improve blood flow. This stretching damages the vessels and eventually reduces the ability of the kidneys to filter out wastes and excess water. If insufficient fluid is filtered from the blood, blood pressure may increase even more, creating a dangerous cycle.

Glomerulonephritis (GN)

Glomerulonephritis (GN), sometimes more simply called *nephritis*, is a kidney disorder caused by damage to or scarring of the glomeruli—the kidneys' tiny blood filters. GN can occur on its own, or it can stem from the effects of another condition, such as lupus, an autoimmune disease; certain bacterial infections, such as pyelonephritis (infection of the kidneys resulting from urinary tract infection); or viral infections such as hepatitis B or C. GN can also be hereditary, and sometimes, the cause is unknown.

Regardless of the disorder's origin, if it is associated with severe or prolonged inflammation, glomerulonephritis can cause a permanent decline in your kidneys' filtration ability.

Other Risk Factors

The development of CKD is clearly connected to specific health conditions, as discussed above. However, your chance of receiving this diagnosis is also linked to other factors. For instance, research shows that your risk of CKD is greater if you are a member of the Native American, Pacific Islander, Asian, Hispanic American, or African American population groups. This may be due to the groups' higher rates of diabetes and high blood pressure, the two leading causes of kidney disease. In addition, it has been shown that age and body type can play a part in the onset of kidney problems, with overweight people and individuals over the age of sixty-five having a greater chance of developing the disorder. Finally, your risk of CKD increases if you smoke or have a history of heart disease or cancer.

While some risk factors for developing kidney disease may be within your control, others are genetic and unchangeable, and still others are a matter of chance. Regardless of the issues that may lead you to a CKD diagnosis, there are ways to slow the rate at which kidney function declines. Therefore, it is helpful to be aware of the disease's presence as soon as possible.

HOW IS KIDNEY DISEASE DIAGNOSED?

As you have read, early declines in kidney function are often symptom-free. Therefore, the first sign of kidney trouble may be a surprise reading that shows up in routine blood work. If something in your blood test suggests that kidney disease might be present, your doctor will no doubt look further by performing a comprehensive examination. Such an exam will include a review of your family medical history; your history of smoking and alcohol or drug use; medical procedures such as surgeries and CT scans; your age, weight, and ethnic background; and your specific dietary habits and any medications taken on a regular basis. Your blood pressure will be reviewed, since pressure that is too high can be both a cause and a result of kidney problems. In addition, your workup will likely include the following special testing to help pinpoint whether CKD is present.

Blood Testing

If kidney disease is suspected, measures of certain substances in your blood will be checked to determine kidney function. The first measure, your *eGFR*, short for *estimated glomerular filtration rate*, shows how efficiently your kidneys are removing wastes from your body. The higher your eGFR, the better your kidneys are working. While eGFR greater than 90mL/min is considered normal, many labs simply report an eGFR greater than 60 mL/min because GFR estimation is not accurate at a near-normal range. For instance, although an eGFR between 60 and 120 milliliters of blood filtered per minute (mL/min) indicates normal or nearly normal function, other findings may still point to the existence of CKD. If you have an eGFR of 95 mL/min but have structural damage to your kidneys or protein or blood in your urine, for example, you may have CKD. An eGFR below 60 mL/min suggests that your kidneys' filtration ability is moderately to significantly impaired. When you read about the stages of kidney disease (see page 21), you'll see how important it is for your doctor to establish your eGFR and why this measure will be closely monitored throughout the course of your treatment.

Your level of *creatinine* will also be measured during blood testing. Creatinine, a material that results from everyday muscle activity, is disposed of in the urine by healthy kidneys but builds up in the blood if there's a problem with kidney function. In adults, normal levels of creatinine range between .5 to 1.2 milligrams per deciliter (mg/dL). Higher levels indicate a problem with your kidneys' ability to filter blood.

Additionally, your level of *blood urea nitrogen (BUN)* will be checked. BUN is produced by the breakdown of food protein and is normally eliminated in the urine as part of a waste product called *urea*. A BUN level in the 6 to 20 mg/dL range is considered normal, but this level will rise as the kidneys lose their filtering ability. Often, the BUN level is used in combination with the creatinine level for the most accurate assessment of kidney function.

Urine Testing

When kidneys are healthy, only tiny, virtually undetectable amounts of protein pass out of the kidneys and into the urine. But when kidneys begin to lose function, they become unable to keep protein in the blood, causing larger amounts of protein to appear in the urine—a condition known as *proteinuria* or *albuminuria*. (Albumin is one of the first proteins to pass into the urine when kidney problems develop.) This may signal the existence of kidney problems even when your blood filtration ability, as indicated by your eGFR, is within normal limits. The presence of red and white blood cells—also normally not found in urine—can also signal kidney disease.

For the protein urine test, a random sample of urine may be tested, or you may be asked to collect your urine for twenty-four hours. Nowadays, your doctor usually estimates the amount of protein in the urine by looking at the *urine protein to creatinine ratio (UPCR)*. The normal protein to creatinine ratio is less than 0.2 gram of protein per gram of creatinine. This is basically the same as having 0.2 gram of protein in the urine per day. A problematic range of urinary protein is greater than 3.5 grams per gram of creatinine and is the same as having 3.5 grams of protein in the urine. Your urine will also be viewed under a microscope for the presence of red blood cells. Values of three or more red cells in the urine may indicate kidney disease.

If the results of your urine test suggest kidney trouble, your doctor may decide that further evaluation is needed.

Other Diagnostic Testing

Depending on your medical history, blood levels, and urinalysis outcome, your doctor may order an imaging test of your kidneys such as ultrasound, a CT scan, or even an MRI. These tests are helpful, because they offer an actual look at the condition of these organs. The information provided by an imaging test can help your doctor identify size abnormalities, structural problems, or blockages. Occasionally, a kidney biopsy may also be requested. This test involves examining small pieces of kidney tissue under a microscope to pinpoint the type of disease that is present.

As you already know, many people with CKD have no symptoms until the disease is well established. Therefore, performing blood and urine tests to check for decreasing renal function is essential to making a timely diagnosis, and an imaging test or biopsy can yield additional important information. Whatever your personal series of tests entails, the results will tell your doctor three important things: whether CKD is present, what the cause of the disease may be, and to what extent your kidney function has declined.

WHAT ARE THE STAGES OF KIDNEY DISEASE?

As you read in Chapter One, your kidneys contain many tiny blood vessels—glomeruli—that continually cleanse your blood. If your kidneys' filtration ability decreases, fluid and wastes begin to build up in the blood rather than exiting your body through the urine. This eventually leads to chemical imbalances and creates problems with other body systems, which can further damage your kidneys and make you feel unwell. Left alone, declining kidney function can become a serious health threat.

With this in mind, the medical community has identified five stages of chronic kidney disease that range from mild to very advanced. The stage of your kidney disease is mainly established using your eGFR, although urine findings and other information about existing kidney abnormalities, your general health, and your family history can play a part. Establishing the stage of your CKD tells you and your doctor the extent to which your kidney function has decreased. It also helps to pinpoint the course of action needed to halt or slow the progress of your condition. Table 2.1 presents a concise look at the five stages of kidney disease and the declines in eGFR and kidney function associated with each. A more detailed description of each stage appears below the table.

Table 2.1   The Five Stages of Chronic Kidney Disease

Stage	Description	Estimated Glomerular Filtration Rate (eGFR)
Stage 1	Normal or high eGFR, with evidence of kidney damage shown by protein and/or blood in urine or by ultrasound, CT scan, or MRI.	90 mL/min or higher
Stage 2	Mild reduction in eGFR, with small amounts of protein and/or blood in urine.	60 to 89 mL/min
Stage 3	Moderate reduction in eGFR, with kidney-related conditions such as anemia or heart and blood vessel disease.	30 to 59 mL/min
Stage 4	Severe reduction in eGFR, with an increase in the number and severity of kidney-related conditions.	15 to 29 mL/min
Stage 5	End-stage renal disease (ESRD), also referred to as kidney failure, with the need for dialysis or kidney transplant.	Less than 15 mL/min

Stage 1 kidney disease is often discovered by accident. In this stage, the possibility of kidney damage may arise through urine test results, knowledge of a genetic condition, or your personal medical history. It can also come from visual evidence of kidney abnormalities as provided by an imaging test. In Stage 1, renal function remains within a normal range and the eGFR measures at 90 mL/min or higher. There are usually no symptoms, and the disease is considered to be *mild* at this point.

Kidney disease in *Stage 2* is also symptom-free in many cases. This stage of CKD is characterized by minimally reduced kidney function as shown by the eGFR, which ranges from 60 to 89 mL/min. There may also be one or more of the same indicators of kidney damage described in Stage 1. While kidney damage has progressed in Stage 2, the disease is still classified as *mild*.

In *Stage 3* CKD, kidney function is increasingly reduced as compared with earlier stages. A lessening in the kidneys' filtration ability leads to a decrease in eGFR of 30 to 59 mL/min. There may also be unpleasant symptoms—such as fatigue and tissue swelling—as a result of the buildup of toxins. (See the inset on page 25 for further signs and symptoms.) In addition, the appearance of kidney disease-related conditions such as high blood pressure or low red blood cell count, commonly referred to as *anemia,* may indicate that other body systems are being affected by declining kidney function. Stage 3 disease is classified as *moderate.*

Stage 4 kidney disease is characterized by severely reduced organ function. A significant decline in the kidneys' filtering ability is indicated by an eGFR between 15 and 29 mL/min. CKD symptoms often increase in number and severity at this point, and complications such as bone disease and heart disease are not unusual. In Stage 4, health conditions suggest an eventual outcome of complete organ failure. Kidney disease at this point is considered to be *advanced.*

Stage 5 CKD is so severe that it is called *end-stage renal disease* (*ESRD*). Other terms for this stage of disease are *kidney failure* and *established renal failure.* Stage 5's eGFR of lower than 15 mL/min shows that the kidneys are barely working and can no longer remove wastes, regulate blood pressure, or perform other tasks crucial to a person's health. Dialysis or a kidney transplant is needed if a patient is to survive. Stage 5 disease is considered to be *very advanced.*

As you see, your doctor is able to determine the stage of your CKD based on your eGFR, your blood and urine tests, and other evidence of kidney damage. Only after establishing the stage can your physician choose a treatment plan. CKD is considered a progressive disease, meaning that any damage that has occurred to your kidneys cannot be undone and tends to get worse over time. However, the condition can be treated effectively. It is possible to delay or even halt the progress of the disease into Stage 3, and the symptoms of kidney disease can be managed beyond that. For that reason, from the moment of diagnosis, a doctor's care is extremely important.

HOW IS KIDNEY DISEASE TREATED?

The overall goal of treatment for CKD is to prevent or slow the further decline of renal function. Regardless of the stage of your disease, it is always advisable to see a kidney specialist, or *nephrologist,* so that you will get the guidance that you need. Studies show that the earlier a patient is referred to a nephrologist, the better the outcome. Your doctor will monitor your kidney function through regular blood and urine testing; adjust your diet to ensure that you are getting the nutrients you need without placing a strain on your kidneys; prescribe medication, if necessary; and manage CKD symptoms and related health problems, such as high blood pressure and diabetes. Lifestyle modifications will be suggested to prevent secondary illnesses and protect your general health, and you will probably be offered help in dealing with the emotional aspects of chronic illness. If and when your CKD progresses to Stage 4, you will begin to learn about the options that will be available to you if artificial filtration—dialysis— becomes necessary. If your general health permits, you may also be told about the possibility of kidney transplant.

Often, CKD management plans utilize a team approach that combines your nephrologist's training and experience with the expertise of other health and wellness professionals. Your healthcare team may include a renal dietitian, who will provide nutritional information,

The Signs and Symptoms of Progressing Kidney Disease

While it isn't unusual for CKD to go unnoticed for a while, the disease's progress is often signaled by a slow development of symptoms that can culminate in what doctors call *uremic symptoms*—that is, signs that kidney function is declining and unfiltered wastes are building up in your body. Once uremic symptoms develop, patients are likely to need dialysis to clear the poisons from the blood. Signs and symptoms of kidney disease may include:

- ☐ **Fatigue, lack of energy, or changes in sleep patterns.** Poor kidney function may mean that your blood doesn't contain enough oxygen because of insufficient red blood cells (anemia). You may feel tired or weak much of the time, but napping to restore energy can interfere with nighttime sleep.

- ☐ **Dizziness or difficulty concentrating.** Lower levels of blood oxygen mean that less oxygen is reaching your brain. This can sometimes cause dizziness and also make it hard to focus on tasks or conversations.

- ☐ **Feeling chilled.** Low blood oxygen can also cause you to feel chronically chilled.

- ☐ **Flank pain.** Some people with kidney problems experience pain on the same side as the affected kidney.

- ☐ **Muscle cramping, especially at night.** An imbalance in fluid and electrolytes like sodium, potassium, and magnesium can cause muscles to cramp painfully.

- ☐ **Poor appetite, digestive problems, and nausea.** As blood chemical levels become unbalanced, food may lose its appeal or begin to taste metallic. You may experience frequent hiccups caused by increasing levels of blood toxins and certain medications. In addition, your stomach may feel upset and you may experience nausea.

- ☐ **Changing urinary habits.** As the kidneys become less efficient in making urine, you may experience frequent urination, the need to urinate during the night, or foamy urine.

☐ **Swelling of the tissues (edema).** As the kidneys become less able to remove extra fluid, fluids build up in the body, causing swelling in the extremities (your hands, ankles, and feet) and puffiness around the eyes.

☐ **Difficulty controlling blood pressure.** A buildup of fluids and an inability to filter out excess sodium can make it difficult to control blood pressure.

☐ **Headaches.** One symptom of the condition called *renal hypertension*—high blood pressure caused by kidney disease—is headache.

☐ **Itchy skin (sometimes called pruritis).** Increasing levels of unfiltered wastes in your blood can cause your skin to feel unusually dry and extremely itchy.

It's helpful to think of CKD symptoms in terms of degrees. The appearance of the symptoms described above, together with irregular blood and urine findings, generally means that disease is preventing the kidneys from adequately filtering the blood and performing other important functions. Additional symptoms may appear as kidney disease advances; however, the focus of this book is on taking action to avoid that outcome. Since CKD symptoms are manageable, be sure to tell your doctor if you experience one of the conditions discussed above.

review and alter your diet when needed, and help you follow important nutritional recommendations. You may also have a counselor who will assist you in coping emotionally with CKD and help you deal with any important decisions that have to be made along the way. And if you decide to pursue complementary treatments such as chiropractic or acupuncture, you may work with professionals in those fields, as well.

YOUR ROLE IN MANAGING YOUR KIDNEY DISEASE

As you can see, the management of CKD is many-sided and requires a good deal of attention. While your healthcare team will be made up of a range of experts, the goal will be for them to complement one another and remain mindful of your primary treatment goal: maintaining kidney function. As you may realize, the overall effectiveness of any management plan often comes down to how thoroughly its guidelines are followed, and this makes your personal role in safeguarding your kidneys a critical one. Fortunately, there are a number of ways in which you can contribute to the success of your CKD therapy.

If you are a smoker, for instance, you can take immediate steps to stop. Besides its well-known cancer risk, smoking has a toxic effect on your body's systems and can lead to kidney inflammation. You can also monitor your weight carefully and work to shed any extra pounds. Excess weight increases the risk of a number of health conditions and places an unnecessary strain on your kidneys. Along these lines, you can resolve to get some form of exercise each day. Besides helping with weight control, regular exercise improves your overall fitness, minimizes stress, and contributes to healthier bones and muscles. Additionally, you can make it a priority to get an appropriate amount of sleep—at least seven to nine hours a night. Getting the sleep you need can refresh, restore, and regenerate your body. (For more lifestyle-related tips, see page 87.)

In addition to the general steps you can take to improve your well-being, discussed above, you can make the decision to be an active member of your healthcare team. Make the members of your team aware of new symptoms or changes in how you feel, and seek their advice before you reduce, stop, or start taking a medication or supplement. Share with them all aspects of your healthcare, and be sure to tell them if you receive unusual medical news from another doctor or are scheduled for an invasive procedure such as surgery. Given the impact of CKD on the whole body, it's important that the professionals who manage your condition have all of the facts about your health. Lastly, you can resolve to cooperate with your team's professional advice and adhere to the diet that will be created for you. As you will see, eating the right foods and carefully avoiding or consuming only limited amounts of other foods is essential to safeguarding kidney function.

IN CONCLUSION

As CKD progresses, it eventually triggers signs within your body that a serious problem exists. You will have the best chance of halting or slowing kidney damage during the early stages of CKD—Stages 1 through 3. But even after the disease has progressed to a later stage, there is much that you and your healthcare team can do to relieve symptoms and improve your overall health. Always keep in mind that many aspects of your condition and the way you feel rest in your own hands. That's why it's vital for you to take an active role in your healthcare by learning all you can about kidney disease, making lifestyle choices with your health in mind, and heeding the recommendations of your team of experts.

You will no doubt find that a large part of your treatment plan involves nutrition. As you'll see in Chapter 3, your goal is to take in the nutrients you need for good health while, as CKD progresses, limiting or avoiding foods that can contribute to a dangerous accumulation of waste products and fluids. By arming yourself with the information that follows, you'll build a nutritional knowledge base that will guide you in following your recommended diet and prove helpful in managing both chronic kidney disease and any related conditions, such as diabetes and hypertension.

3

Nutrition and Chronic Kidney Disease

Nutrition experts agree that a healthy diet should contain nutrient-rich foods that provide the body with vitamins, minerals, protein, and other essential components of good health. But as you already know, a diet that is considered healthy for the average person can create serious problems if you have impaired kidney function. In fact, some of the nutrients that an individual without CKD can and should eat in abundance must be severely limited in some CKD diets.

This chapter provides important information about special dietary considerations for the individual with chronic kidney disease. You'll discover why published dietary guidelines may not apply to people with kidney problems, learn about specific nutrients that may have to be restricted in your diet, and become familiar with the foods that are the best choices when CKD is present. In addition, you'll become aware of factors that can influence your appetite and nutritional needs throughout your treatment or for extended periods of time.

PUTTING STANDARD DIETARY RECOMMENDATIONS INTO PERSPECTIVE

Many of us grew up in families that prepared meals in line with the recommended dietary guidelines of the time. You see, for more than a century, the United States Department of Agriculture (USDA) has published nutritional guides, originally to make sure that everyone enjoyed a balanced diet that included foods from all "food groups"— and, therefore, included all nutrients—and later to ensure that everyone's diet focused on the foods that promoted optimal health. From 1943 to 1956, the USDA recommended the "Basic Seven" food groups. From 1956 until 1992, the "Basic Four" were advised. The Food Guide Pyramid, introduced in 1992, advocated serving numbers and sizes so that the American diet would contain more of the foods considered vital to good health and less of the foods viewed as being nutrient-poor or even harmful. This was succeeded by MyPyramid (2005) and MyPlate (2011). The United States government also publishes a collection of nutritional recommendations called *Dietary Guidelines for Americans.*

In addition to providing the broad dietary suggestions just discussed, over the years, the government has recommended specific amounts of important nutrients in the form of the Recommended Daily Allowances (RDAs) and the Dietary Reference Intakes (DRIs). The intention of these recommendations has been to prevent nutritional deficiencies and/or reduce the risk of chronic disease.

Finally, as you are probably well aware, health experts have endorsed various eating plans—the Mediterranean diet, for instance— as a means of optimizing health and reducing common disorders such as obesity, heart disease, and diabetes.

The nutritional guidelines and specific recommendations that have been provided over the years have addressed real dietary problems and, in some cases, have reflected important scientific research. While a good deal of these recommendations have been valuable, even the most up-to-date guidelines aren't right for everyone. People with CKD have very special nutritional needs that make it essential to follow the diet recommended by their healthcare team. Your healthcare team will urge you to consume adequate amounts of the nutrients you need to protect your health. Just as important, they will guide you in avoiding foods that contain large amounts of the substances that can build up to dangerous levels in an individual whose kidney function is impaired. The following discussions go into greater detail about the nutrients that often must be limited on a renal diet.

COMMON DIETARY COMPONENTS AND CKD

As you'll recall from Chapter 2, weakened kidneys cannot efficiently filter excess chemical and waste materials from the blood. That's why a standard diet isn't advisable as damage to your kidney progresses, because your meals would likely provide too much of the substances that your kidneys are no longer able to handle, causing dangerous levels of chemicals to accumulate in the blood and worsening kidney damage by placing a strain on the organs. Slowing or stopping declining kidney function is an essential goal when CKD is present, so it's extremely important to avoid foods that burden the kidneys. In some cases, this means eliminating or severely restricting foods that are generally thought of as being healthful. For instance, milk, considered by most people to be a wholesome drink, is often restricted when kidney disease is present because it is high in phosphorus and potassium—two minerals that ailing kidneys cannot properly filter out of the blood.

As you have already read, your kidney health may change over time. Your healthcare team will monitor your kidney function at each office visit and, based on your test results, will make specific dietary recommendations that are right for you at that time. Their professional advice, which is aimed at keeping your CKD from getting worse, should be followed closely. The nutritional information presented in the pages that follow will help you understand the importance of the dietary guidelines you receive from your team. It will also guide you in choosing the most kidney-friendly foods and beverages available.

Protein

Proteins have been referred to as the building blocks of life because the body needs protein to build and maintain all body cells and tissues. This nutrient also provides your body with energy, controls body functions, transports certain molecules, helps with digestion, prevents infection, and more. Many Americans, though, eat much more of this nutrient than needed. This can lead to a number of problems, including kidney disease, as too much protein places a strain on the kidneys as they struggle to expel the extra nitrogen contained in the food. As you can imagine, this is a particular problem for people whose kidney function has decreased due to CKD.

If you have kidney disease that is in Stage 1, 2, or 3, the general recommendation for daily protein intake is 0.75 g/kg (grams per kilogram) of body weight. In later stages of CKD, the recommendation for protein drops to 0.6 g/kg. You can find your weight in kilograms by dividing your weight in pounds by 2.2. So, for example, a 176-pound individual weighs 80 kg. (176 ÷ 2.2 = 80.) The recommended amount of protein for this individual in early-stage CKD would be about 60 g per day. (80 × .75 = 60.) Your personal circumstances may call for a variation in this formula, of course. Your

Keeping Your Food Safe

Everyone would benefit from eating fresh foods that are free of additives and other contaminants, but this becomes even more important for the individual with chronic kidney disease, whose body is less able to rid itself of toxins and handle harmful foodborne bacteria. That's why you should keep the following points in mind when selecting and preparing foods for the individual with CKD.

☐ **Avoid food additives.** Thickeners, flavoring, coloring, preservatives, stabilizers, antioxidants, and even hormones are put in foods to make them look and taste better or to preserve freshness or smell. These chemical additions can take a toll on someone with CKD. While the Food and Drug Administration (FDA) places limits on the quantities of additives used in processed and packaged foods and beverages, their regulations have been created with the average person in mind. Remember that these limits may not hold true for people whose kidney function is compromised, and that you should always check ingredients lists for the presence of added chemicals. (To learn more about the additives in beverages, see the inset on page 54.) Of course, the best alternative is to buy fresh foods and prepare them yourself.

healthcare team will guide you in establishing a daily protein goal that is right for you.

It's important to know that there are many sources of protein—some animal-based and some plant-based—and that some proteins may be better for you than others, depending upon your health status. The animal-based proteins found in eggs, meat, fish, and poultry contain a full complement of *essential amino acids,* the basic building blocks of protein that can be supplied only through diet. Because these foods are lower in phosphorus and potassium than dairy foods and plant-based proteins such as nuts and seeds, they produce fewer waste products. When choosing animal proteins, it's better for your general health to focus on leaner, lower-fat selections, such as skinless white meat chicken, fish, and egg whites or whole eggs combined

☐ **Choose foods that are as free as possible from pesticides and environmental contaminants.** Whenever possible, buy organic meats, fruits, and vegetables—foods produced without pesticides and other chemicals. If organic produce is not available, be sure to scrub fruits and vegetables thoroughly under running water to wash away chemical residue.

☐ **Buy the freshest food available—and use it while it's still fresh.** Always purchase and serve the freshest food you can find. Make it a practice to check the expiration and "sell by" dates when selecting a product. If you choose to purchase a frozen item, avoid frost-covered or unusually soft packages. This can indicate that the product may have been thawed and refrozen, which could lead to bacterial contamination. When you get your foods home from the market, promptly transfer them to your refrigerator or freezer as necessary.

☐ **Follow food safety practices when preparing a meal.** Thoroughly wash your hands before preparing a meal, and keep utensils and chopping boards clean. To avoid cross-contamination, keep raw meat and poultry from touching other foods during preparation, and use different chopping boards for different foods. Cook foods thoroughly, and promptly refrigerate leftovers once you've finished eating.

Eggs and CKD

Anyone who's interested in following a healthful diet may be more than a little confused about eggs, which have received both good and bad press over the years. Are eggs a rich source of nutrients, or are they a dangerous source of cholesterol? Most important, do eggs have a place in a CKD diet?

If you turn to the recipe section, which begins on page 97, you'll find that a number of the recipes in this book do contain eggs. That's because eggs are a great source of protein. But most of our egg recipes combine whole eggs with egg whites or egg substitutes. That's because the egg yolk—while it contains vitamins A, D, E, and K, as well as a host of other nutrients—contains cholesterol and phosphorus, which have to be limited in a good many CKD diets. Egg whites provide protein without the cholesterol and phosphorus, but also without the healthful fat-soluble vitamins found in the yolk.

The bottom line is that eggs are a valuable food, but the safest way to enjoy their benefits is to eat them only three to four days a week and to prepare your dishes with a combination of whole eggs and egg whites or egg substitutes. This strategy will provide you with the full nutrients of the egg yolk without increasing your cardiovascular risk or providing more phosphorus than your body can handle.

with egg whites. (To learn about incorporating eggs into your diet, see the inset above.) Avoid processed meats, as almost all processed foods provide too much sodium and are "enhanced" with phosphorus. Fresh, unprocessed foods are always best.

While animal proteins provide complete amino acids, they can have a downside. These proteins can place a strain on the kidneys and speed their decline. And, of course, they can provide too much saturated fat for people with certain health conditions. For these reasons, your healthcare team may advise you to limit meats and eat a variety of plant foods that, in combination, can provide complete proteins and be gentler on your kidneys. Your team may especially emphasize the importance of higher-protein plant foods, such as tofu, lentils, and beans. Be aware that these foods, too, can have disadvantages. Some of the highest-protein plant sources are also high in phosphorus, potassium, or both. Therefore, the intake of some plant protein sources—lentils, for instance—may be restricted, especially if blood levels of phosphorus or potassium are high. That's why getting the amount of protein you need, without getting too much and without upsetting your blood chemical levels, can be a balancing act. Moderation and knowledge of your personal nutritional needs are vital.

Below, you'll find a list of high-quality proteins; a list of protein sources that are good, but are recommended with reservations; and a list of protein sources whose consumption should generally be restricted by people with CKD. It can't be overemphasized that when choosing proteins, you must seek the dietary advice of your health-care team. Your doctor and dietitian will guide you in selecting the protein sources that best fit your specific health needs.

The Best Dietary Sources of Protein

❏ Eggs, especially egg whites, a combination of whole eggs and extra whites, or egg substitute

❏ Fish

❏ Meats, such as lean beef and pork

❏ Poultry (skinless), such as chicken and turkey breast

❏ Tofu

Protein Sources Recommended with Reservations

❏ Beans, especially chickpeas (chickpeas are relatively low in potassium)

❏ Grains, such as quinoa and bulgur wheat

❏ Lentils

Protein Sources That Should be Limited

❏ Dairy products such as milk, cheese, and yogurt

❏ Organ meats, such as liver

❏ Processed meats, such as cold cuts

❏ Baked beans with added sugar or pork

How to Read a Food Label
Tips for People with Chronic Kidney Disease (CKD)

If you have CKD, you may need to limit some nutrients in your diet such as sodium, phosphorus, or potassium. You should limit saturated and trans fats, too. Read the food label to help make healthy food choices for your kidneys.

- Check the Nutrition Facts label for sodium.

- Check the ingredient list for added phosphorus and potassium.

- Look for claims on the label, like "low saturated fat" or "sodium free."

What Should I Look for on the Nutrition Facts Label?

Look for **sodium** on the Nutrition Facts label. Some Nutrition Facts labels will list **phosphorus** and **potassium**, too, but they do not have to.

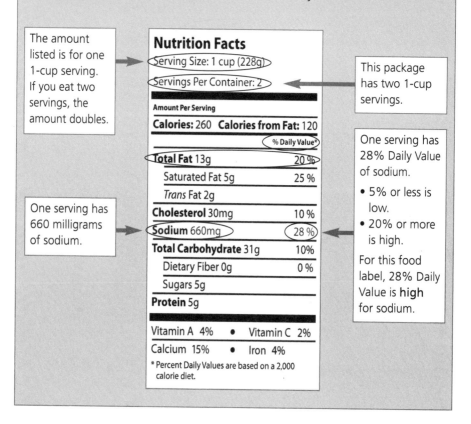

The amount listed is for one 1-cup serving. If you eat two servings, the amount doubles.

This package has two 1-cup servings.

One serving has 660 milligrams of sodium.

One serving has 28% Daily Value of sodium.
- 5% or less is low.
- 20% or more is high.

For this food label, 28% Daily Value is **high** for sodium.

Nutrition Facts

Serving Size: 1 cup (228g)

Servings Per Container: 2

Amount Per Serving

Calories: 260 **Calories from Fat:** 120

% Daily Value*

Total Fat 13g	20 %
Saturated Fat 5g	25 %
Trans Fat 2g	
Cholesterol 30mg	10 %
Sodium 660mg	28 %
Total Carbohydrate 31g	10%
Dietary Fiber 0g	0 %
Sugars 5g	
Protein 5g	

Vitamin A 4%	•	Vitamin C 2%
Calcium 15%	•	Iron 4%

* Percent Daily Values are based on a 2,000 calorie diet.

What Should I Look for on the Ingredient List?

1. Look for **phosphorus**, or for words with PHOS, on the ingredient list. Many packaged foods have phosphorus. Choose a different food when the ingredient list has PHOS on the label.

> **Ingredients:** Rehydrated potatoes (Water, Potatoes, Sodium acid pyro**phos**phate), Beef (Beef, Water, Salt, Sodium **phos**phate), Wine . . .
> *This ingredient list shows that the food has added phosphorus.*

2. Look for **potassium** on the ingredient list. For example, potassium chloride can be used in place of salt in some packaged foods, like canned soups and tomato products. Limit foods with potassium on the ingredient list.

> **Ingredients:** Tomato juice, Vegetable juice blend, **Potassium** chloride, Sugar, Magnesium, Salt, Vitamin C (Ascorbic acid), Citric acid, Spice extract, Flavoring, Disodium inosinate, Disodium guanylate.
> *This ingredient list shows that the food has added potassium.*

Did You Know?

Ingredients are listed in order of the amount in the food. The food has the most of the first ingredient on the list, and the least of the last ingredient on the list.

Look for Claims on Food Packages to Help You Find Foods:

Lower in Saturated/Trans Fat	Lower in Sodium
• Saturated fat free	• Sodium free
• Low saturated fat	• Very low sodium
• Less saturated fat	• Low sodium
• Trans fat free	• Reduced salt

* Reprinted courtesy of the National Kidney Disease Education Program of the National Institutes of Health (visit www.nkdep.nih.gov).

Potassium

Potassium helps to keep your heart, muscles, and nerves healthy and in good working order. In addition, potassium helps to regulate your blood pressure and maintain the proper balance of fluids and chemicals in your blood. Like other minerals, potassium comes from the food you eat and can accumulate in your body if you consume too much. This isn't a problem for healthy kidneys, which filter out excess potassium and release it from the body in the urine. When kidney function declines, however, potassium buildup can eventually reach unsafe levels.

While potassium recommendations for people with kidney problems vary according to the stage of the disorder, in general, people with moderate or severe CKD should consume around 2,700 mg of the mineral per day. That number may drop to 2,000 mg or less in late stages of the disease before dialysis begins. It is worth noting that certain medications and concurrent health problems can lead to potassium levels that are dangerously low and may require increased dietary potassium or even potassium pills. As with other nutrients that must be watched when managing kidney problems, your healthcare team will use your blood work to determine exactly how much potassium is right for you.

The Dangers of Star Fruit

While some fruits, such as bananas, may have to be limited on a CKD diet, there is one fruit that must be completely avoided—star fruit. Also known as carambola, this star-shaped produce is not dangerous to people with normal kidney function, but it is poisonous for people whose kidney function is impaired.

Star fruit contains a neurotoxin known as caramboxin, and when kidney disease is present, the body is unable to eliminate this toxin from the body. Within hours of consumption, caramboxin can enter the brain and cause symptoms that include persistent hiccups, vomiting, hearing impairment, confusion, anxiety, numbness, seizures, and even death. The bottom line is that whatever your stage of CKD, you must avoid this sweet poison.

Leaching Vegetables to Reduce Potassium

Vegetables are an important part of a healthy diet, but some vegetables are high in potassium. The steps below explain how to reduce the potassium content of beets, carrots, rutabagas, sweet potatoes, white potatoes, and winter squash, potentially increasing the portion size you can eat. The leaching process also works for frozen greens. As with any change in your diet, you should consult your healthcare team before consuming leached vegetables. Your dietitian can recommend the appropriate serving sizes for your health needs.

1. Peel and slice root vegetables to $1/8$-inch thicknesses. Thaw frozen vegetables and drain of any liquid.

2. Rinse the prepared vegetables in warm water for a few seconds.

3. Place the vegetables in a large bowl, and top with ten times the amount of warm water as vegetables. (For instance, add ten cups of warm water to one cup of sliced carrots.) Soak for at least two hours. If you soak the vegetables longer, change the water every four hours.

4. Drain the water from the bowl and rinse the vegetables again in fresh warm water.

5. Cook the vegetables, using five times the amount of water as vegetables. (For instance, one cup of sliced carrots should be cooked in five cups of water.) Drain the water after cooking, and serve.

It can be tricky to monitor your intake of potassium, because manufacturers currently are not required to list this mineral on Nutrition Facts labels for their food products. (To learn more about using the Nutrition Facts label, see the inset on page 36.) Potassium products may be found among a food's ingredients, though, so it's important to get in the habit of reading this list. You'll be better able to avoid too much potassium if you limit items whose ingredients include components with the word "potassium" in their names, such as "potassium chloride." Also bear in mind that traditional dietary staples such as potatoes, tomatoes, and dairy products tend to be high in potassium, and that the mineral is present in many other foods, as well as nutritional supplements and medications.

It is possible to remove some of the potassium from certain fresh vegetables, which may enable you to eat them in larger portions. The inset on page 39 guides you in doing this. You can also lower your potassium intake by seasoning your foods only with spices and herbs, because salt substitutes (which help you avoid sodium) are high in potassium; and by draining the liquid from canned fruits and vegetables. Finally, portion size is a crucial consideration. Because too large a serving of even a low-potassium food can provide more of the mineral than your kidneys can handle, it is wise to stick to $\frac{1}{2}$-cup portions. Your healthcare team will determine exactly how much potassium you should take in by reviewing your blood work on an ongoing basis. Below, you will find lists of low-potassium foods, as well as high-potassium foods that should be avoided or eaten on a very limited basis. These lists will help you plan meals and choose snacks that can keep your potassium level within a safe range.

Low-Potassium Food Sources

❏ Apples

❏ Asparagus

❏ Berries

❏ Bread, other than whole grain

❏ Broccoli, raw

❏ Carrots, cooked

❏ Cauliflower

❏ Celery

❏ Cherries

❏ Corn

❏ Cranberries

❏ Cucumbers

❏ Garlic

❏ Grapes

❏ Green beans

❏ Lettuce

❏ Onions

❏ Pasta and noodles, other than whole grain

❏ Peaches

❏ Peppers

❏ Pineapple

❏ Plums

❏ Tangerines

❏ White rice

❏ Yellow summer squash

❏ Zucchini squash

High-Potassium Foods to Limit or Avoid

❏ Acorn squash

❏ Apricots

❏ Avocados

❏ Bananas

❏ Beans

❏ Beets

❏ Broccoli, cooked

❏ Brown rice

❏ Brussels sprouts

❏ Carrots, raw, and carrot juice

❏ Chocolate

❏ Clams

❏ Dark leafy greens

❏ Dates

❏ Figs

❏ Kiwi

❏ Lentils

❏ Mangos

❏ Melons

❏ Milk, cheese, yogurt, and other dairy products

❏ Mushrooms

❏ Nectarines

❏ Nuts

❏ Okra

❏ Oranges and orange juice

❏ Peanuts

❏ Pomegranates

❏ Potatoes, white or sweet

❏ Prunes and prune juice

❏ Raisins

❏ Rutabagas

❏ Salt substitutes that contain potassium

❏ Sardines

❏ Soy milk, cheese, and yogurt

❏ Tomatoes and tomato juice

❏ Wheat germ

❏ Whole-grain bread

❏ Whole-grain pasta and noodles

❏ Winter squash

Sodium

As discussed in Chapter 1, sodium (salt) is very important to the regulation of blood pressure and the balance of fluids in your body. Sodium also helps your cells absorb nutrients and assists with muscle function. Very high or low levels of the mineral can create health problems, and it's especially important to monitor your sodium intake when kidney problems exist. As you already know, impaired kidneys cannot filter out large amounts of sodium, and the resulting buildup of this mineral can lead to increased blood pressure, fluid retention, and other serious problems.

It is generally suggested that someone with CKD or high blood pressure consume 1,500 to 2,000 mg of sodium each day to get the amount the body needs and yet prevent excess sodium from accumulating. However, meeting this goal can be a challenge. After all, sodium is widely used in foods and beverages and can also be found in some over-the-counter medications and supplements. Your healthcare team will pay close attention to your blood sodium and fluid levels and advise you regarding the maximum amount of sodium you can have in your diet. In addition, you can take important steps on your own to limit your sodium consumption.

First, it helps to avoid canned, processed, and packaged foods in favor of fresh fruits and vegetables and lean meats. If prepared foods must be used, look for salt-free and low- or reduced-sodium products. If feasible, eliminate additional salt by rinsing the food with water or pouring off packaging liquid. You can also switch from table salt to other seasonings such as lemon, ginger, herbs, fresh onion, or hot sauce. While salt substitutes are available, most of these contain other problematic ingredients such as potassium and should be avoided. Additionally, monitor the sodium content of the food you eat by reading Nutrition Facts labels. (See the inset on page 36.) Also, check ingredient lists for the word "sodium" as part of an ingredient name—as in "sodium chloride," for instance—as this indicates that extra sodium has been added to the product. To help you plan meals that limit the sodium in your diet, both high-sodium and low-sodium food lists are presented below.

Low-Sodium Food Sources

❑ Dishes made with fresh meat and vegetables but no salt, including casseroles, soups, sauces, and salad dressings

❑ Eggs

❑ Fresh beef, fish, pork, and poultry

❑ Fresh fruits and vegetables, including garlic and onion

❑ Lemon juice

❑ Low- or no-sodium seasoning blends

High-Sodium Foods to Avoid

- ❏ Bouillon cubes
- ❏ Canned and dehydrated soups, broths, and gravies
- ❏ Canned vegetables, unless the label specifies "no added salt"
- ❏ Cheese
- ❏ Cured and processed meats, such as cold cuts, bacon, and salami, unless the label specifies "no added salt"
- ❏ Frozen meals
- ❏ Marmite yeast extract
- ❏ Pickled foods such as olives and dill pickles
- ❏ Saltwater crab
- ❏ Snack foods such as chips and pretzels
- ❏ Soy sauce and tamari
- ❏ Table salt

Phosphorus

Working in conjunction with calcium and vitamin D, phosphorus is essential for bone health. It also plays an important role in the body's use of fats and carbohydrates. Like levels of other minerals, the level of phosphorus in your blood is controlled by the kidneys, which normally eliminate excess amounts. Phosphorus levels generally do not rise in early stage CKD, but when the disease progresses into Stage 3, excess phosphorus can't be efficiently filtered and eliminated, causing blood levels of this mineral to rise. Phosphorus levels that are too high can lead to bone pain, bone thinning, fractures, and heart disease. To avoid such problems, your healthcare team will monitor your blood work and, when necessary, will recommend that you limit dietary phosphorus. As time goes on, phosphorus binders such as Tums may be ordered to slow your body's absorption of phosphorus. Generally speaking, phosphorus intake should be limited to 800 to 1,000 mg per day when you have moderate to severe CKD.

Almost all foods contain some phosphorus, but some food items contain a very high amount. For example, chocolate and cola drinks are very high in phosphorus, as are ale, beer, and certain types of seafood. If you've been told to limit your phosphorus intake, it is wise to avoid these foods as much as possible.

Phosphorus, like potassium, is not required to be listed on Nutrition Facts labels, although some companies voluntarily include the content of this mineral. However, components that add phosphorus to a product do have to be listed among the item's ingredients. It's important, therefore, to check ingredient lists for substances with "phos" in their names, such as "sodium phosphate," "phosphoric acid," or "sodium triphosphate," for this indicates the presence of added phosphorus. The inset on page 36 will help you understand more about food labels.

A list of good low-phosphorus food choices is presented below, along with foods that are high in phosphorus content. When selecting foods, it's important to know that dietary phosphorus is found in different forms. *Organic phosphorus,* found in plants and animals, has relatively low absorption by the gastrointestinal tract. Usually, 40 to 60 percent of animal-based phosphorus is absorbed, and 40 to 50 percent of plant-based phosphorus is absorbed. However, up to 100 percent of dietary *inorganic phosphorus*—most of which comes from food preservatives—is absorbed. While this doesn't mean that that you can eat all the phosphorus-rich vegetables you want, it does mean that you should be particularly diligent to avoid processed foods. Remember, too, that when considering low-phosphorus alternatives, you need to be mindful of other components of the foods you choose, such as sodium or potassium, that may lead to different problems if too much is consumed.

Low-Phosphorus Food Sources

❏ Atlantic cod and grouper

❏ Barley, pearled

❏ Beef, lean

❏ Bread, other than whole grain

❏ Catsup, salt-free

❏ Corn flakes or crispy rice cereal

❏ Eggs

❏ Farina and hominy grits

❏ Gelatin

❏ Oysters

❏ Pasta and noodles, other than whole grain

❏ Pork, lean

❏ Poultry (skinless), such as chicken, duck, or turkey breast

❏ Sherbet

❏ Shrimp

❏ Soy milk

❏ White rice

High-Phosphorus Foods to Limit or Avoid

- Beans, including dried, canned, and baked
- Beer and ale
- Bologna
- Bran cereal
- Brewer's yeast
- Brown rice
- Cake
- Canned iced tea
- Caramels
- Chocolate
- Chocolate drinks
- Crayfish
- Dark colas and certain other sodas (check the ingredients list)
- Hot dogs
- Lentils
- Macaroni and cheese
- Meats such as ham that are "enhanced" (injected with water and other ingredients)
- Milk, cheese, yogurt, and other dairy foods
- Nuts and nut butters, including peanut butter
- Organ meats, such as liver
- Pizza
- Processed foods containing preservatives and additives
- Sardines
- Seeds
- Wheat germ
- Whole-grain bread
- Whole-grain pasta and noodles

Calcium

Calcium is necessary for bone health and also helps your heart, muscles, and nerves to function properly. Under normal circumstances, the kidneys turn vitamin D into an active hormone, *calcitriol,* which helps the body absorb dietary calcium into the blood and bones. But when your kidneys aren't working properly, they cannot produce calcitriol, and an insufficient amount of calcium is absorbed by the body. As calcium blood levels fall, the body leaches the mineral out of the bones, which not only weakens the bones but can also cause calcium to

When "Good" Foods Are Bad for You

Over the years, most of us have been told that certain foods are "good" and certain foods are "bad." Usually, the good foods are high in vitamins, minerals, and other nutrients that the body needs, and the bad foods are nutrient-poor. But when you have CKD, some of the foods previously deemed beneficial now must be limited or even avoided.

Let's take rice, for instance. You may know that brown rice is usually considered more healthful than white rice because it retains the nutrient-packed hull and bran, which have been removed from white rice. But among the nutrients that brown rice supplies in higher amounts are potassium and phosphorus—two minerals that many people with CKD must limit because their bodies are unable to filter excess amounts out of the blood. This makes white rice preferable. Similarly, whole-grain breads supply too much phosphorus and potassium for some CKD patients, making white breads a safer choice.

Everybody with chronic kidney disease has different nutritional needs, and these needs can change over time. If you're not sure if or why some foods need to be restricted, ask your doctor or renal dietitian. If you've been told that certain nutrients must be monitored and you need guidance in choosing suitable foods, further help is available from the American Association of Kidney Patients (AAKP), which offers a Nutrition Counter that lists 300 common foods with recommended portion sizes and complete nutrient contents. To download a copy of the Nutrition Counter brochure, visit the AAKP website. (See page 186 of the Resources list.)

be deposited in the blood vessels, where it contributes to heart disease. To make matters worse, some of the best sources of calcium, such as dairy products and calcium-fortified orange juice, are restricted for people with CKD because of high levels of other minerals.

It is generally suggested that people with CKD consume between 1,400 and 1,600 mg of calcium per day, not to exceed 2,000 mg per day. But clearly, CKD not only makes it difficult to take in adequate amounts of this mineral but can also prevent the body from absorbing and using the calcium that is consumed. Your healthcare team will monitor both your bone density and your blood calcium levels to determine the exact calcium intake that is right for you. If your calcium is found to be low, a calcium supplement may be prescribed. Since low calcium can be a sign of vitamin D deficiency, your doctor may prescribe an activated form of vitamin D to aid absorption. Phophorus binders are sometimes necessary to restore the balance between calcium and phosphorus.

If your calcium levels are excessively high, calcium supplements and calcium-based phosphorus binders will be limited or avoided, as will active vitamin D.

Magnesium

The mineral magnesium helps to maintain your heart rhythm, aids normal nerve and muscle function, keeps bones strong, and supports a healthy immune system. It also plays a part in the regulation of your blood sugar and blood pressure. When kidneys are healthy, this mineral is absorbed during digestion and any excess is released in the urine. However, factors associated with kidney disease, such as decreased filtration ability, health complications, medications, and fluctuating levels of other minerals, can lead to magnesium levels that are too high or too low. This, in turn, can cause serious health problems.

The general recommended magnesium intake for people with CKD is 200 mg per day, with bran cereal, nuts, beans, spinach, potatoes, and milk being among the best sources. Unfortunately, magnesium-rich foods are often restricted because they contain other minerals that are problematic when kidney disease is present. In addition, antacids, laxatives, and tap water all contain magnesium, which can make it tricky to monitor your intake of this mineral. By checking your blood work frequently, your healthcare team will be able to advise you as to the precise amount and best sources of magnesium for your health needs.

Fiber

Dietary fiber is a type of carbohydrate that passes through the body undigested. There are two types of fiber—soluble and insoluble.

Soluble fiber dissolves in water and can help lower glucose levels by slowing digestion, and thereby slowing the release of glucose into the blood. It may also help to regulate cholesterol, and, by delaying the emptying of the stomach, it can make you feel fuller, reducing the risk of excess weight. *Insoluble fiber* does not dissolve in water, so it adds bulk to waste, helping it to move more quickly through the digestive system.

Regardless of the health of your kidneys, the daily recommendation for fiber is 21 to 25 g for women and 30 to 38 g for men. Americans in general do not get enough of this healthful substance, and people with chronic kidney disease are hampered by the fact that the best sources of fiber—bran, whole-grain products, vegetables, and fruits—often must be eaten in limited quantities because of high levels of phosphorus and potassium. Your healthcare team will help you increase the fiber in your diet by recommending daily small portions of certain whole fruits, cereals, and breads that are less likely to upset your body's chemical levels. If necessary, a fiber supplement such as Citrucel may be suggested.

Vitamin D

As discussed earlier in the chapter, vitamin D plays a key role in keeping your bones healthy. It has also been suggested that this vitamin helps reduce the risk of heart disease, diabetes, and cancer. Vitamin D has long been called "the sunshine vitamin," but when kidney problems are present and your body struggles to produce the active form of vitamin D you need, sunlight isn't enough. Unfortunately, food may not be too helpful either. Few foods are good natural sources of vitamin D, the best being fatty fish such as bluefish, mackerel, salmon, sardines, and tuna. Other products such as vitamin-D fortified milk and breakfast cereals usually have to be limited by people with CKD because they also contain minerals that can build up to toxic levels. As a result, it isn't unusual for people with kidney problems to have low vitamin D levels and require a supplement.

Your healthcare team will track your vitamin D level through your regular blood work and prescribe a supplement of activated

Tips for Eating Right with CKD

This chapter fills you in on foods that are kidney-protective as well as foods that can place a strain on the kidneys and, perhaps, cause further damage. There's certainly a lot to know, so this inset highlights some of the most important points you should keep in mind as you choose and prepare your foods.

☐ **Be protein picky.** Eat lean, high-quality proteins. Remember that lean animal proteins can help you meet your needs for this valuable nutrient while producing minimal waste products. Although plant-based proteins produce more wastes than animal proteins, they can be gentler on your kidneys—as long as you stay within your potassium and phosphorus limits. Just as important, be sure to remain within your daily protein limits. (See page 31 for more information about protein.)

☐ **Make pure water your go-to beverage.** To avoid potentially harmful levels of sugar and those minerals that can build up to toxic levels—as well as environmental contaminants—choose the purest water available to fill your fluid requirements. (See page 51 for more information.) Then do your best to stay within your daily fluid limits.

☐ **Manage those minerals.** Take heed of any limitations regarding dietary minerals—sodium, potassium, and phosphorus—and choose foods that will allow you to consume healthy amounts of these nutrients.

☐ **Avoid processed foods.** As much as possible, steer clear of processed foods, including canned foods, frozen foods, deli meats, refrigerated prepared foods, bottled beverages (except for water), and the like. These foods are often loaded with unhealthy amounts of sugar, sodium, potassium, phosphorus, chemical additives, and other ingredients that can harm both your kidneys and your general health. Fresh foods prepared with healthy flavorings such as garlic and herbs (no salt!) are always your best bet. If you rely on some processed foods for convenience, look for no-salt-added choices that are additive- and preservative-free.

☐ **Choose nutrient-dense foods.** Focusing on foods that are nutritionally dense—that is, lower in calories and higher in the vitamins and minerals your doctor recommends—is another good strategy. By making nutrient-dense foods the center of your diet, you will consume higher-quality fare that carries less risk of weight gain. Options that are good for people with CKD include skinless chicken and turkey, egg whites, and low-potassium fruits and vegetables, such as fresh cherries and green beans.

☐ **Pay attention to portion size.** Heaping portions can turn healthful food into food that supplies a dangerous amount of minerals, so always keep portion sizes in line with your nutritional limitations. When using processed foods, note that the nutrient counts listed on the Nutrition Facts label are for one serving only. If you exceed this amount, you may get more fat, sodium, potassium, or phosphorus than you bargained for.

☐ **Always listen to your healthcare team.** As we discuss throughout this chapter, your healthcare team—your doctor and/or your renal dietitian—will keep you informed about fluid restrictions as well as limits placed on other nutrients. Choose your diet in keeping with their recommendations, and be aware that their advice may change over time as your health status changes.

vitamin D if levels need to be boosted. Since multivitamins and many calcium supplements contain vitamin D—and multivitamins contain some nutrients that must be consumed only in limited quantities by some people with CKD—be sure to talk to your doctor before taking one of these products. (See the inset on page 52 for more about vitamin supplements.)

Fluids

As you read in Chapter 1, controlling the level of fluid in your body is quite important when you have CKD. It is a tricky undertaking, since kidney problems often lead to decreased filtration and the potential for a buildup of wastes, including excess fluid. If your body retains too much fluid, you can experience symptoms such as weight gain, increased blood pressure, edema (the swelling of tissues), and shortness of breath. Significant fluid buildup can lead to serious heart problems, as well.

Ultimately, your healthcare team will tell you how much fluid you should take in each day and help you determine the best ways to meet your fluid goal. As you try to keep within your limits, remember that your fluid intake comes not only from drinking water and other beverages, but also from other foods that contain water. For instance, fruits and vegetables tend to have high water contents, and water is an ingredient in numerous other foods, such as soups. *Any* fluid you consume, whether in a beverage or in another food, counts as part of your daily fluid intake. Also keep in mind that the sodium you consume has a direct effect on the amount of fluid your body retains, making it critical to limit the sodium in your diet. (See page 41 for more about restricting sodium.)

Naturally, you'll want to make sure that the fluids you do drink are healthy and free of contaminants. Try to fulfill your daily fluid quota with high-quality water, perhaps flavored with a squirt of fresh lime or lemon juice. Drinking water has been known to become tainted by farming or landscaping pesticides, or by chemicals from plumbing materials or nearby industrial sources. Well water can also be subject to contamination by arsenic, toxins, or bacteria. As you might suspect, the presence of such pollutants can play particular havoc with the blood chemical levels and overall health of someone whose kidneys have lost some of their ability to filter out contaminants due to CKD. You should also be aware that additional sodium may be used in exchange for other minerals as a way to decrease water's hardness. It's advisable, therefore, to ask your local water authority for their Consumer Confidence Report, an annual document listing detected levels of regulated contaminants. The report indicates whether any problem exists.

Although the report from your local water authority is valuable, keep in mind that this information is geared for the average person and not someone with reduced kidney function. If you have CKD, you may prefer to cleanse your tap water of pollutants and chemicals with a carbon filter. Better yet, invest in a reverse osmosis filter that removes additional contaminants such as chromium. If you prefer to drink bottled water, be aware that not all companies are completely transparent about the quality of their water. Some companies simply bottle and sell purified tap water. It is wise to check for three facts on a bottle's label before you make your purchase: the location of the water source, the treatment methods used, and whether a water quality report is available online. You can have added confidence in the water's safety if this information is clearly stated. Avoid bottles that contain BPA (bisphenol A), a toxin that can leach into the water.

Vitamin-Mineral Supplements and Chronic Kidney Disease

The body needs a range of vitamins and minerals to function properly. The best way to get these nutrients is by eating a balanced diet, but people with chronic kidney disease often find it hard to obtain the nutrients they need because of poor appetite, necessary dietary restrictions, and other factors. And when dialysis is required, that process, although lifesaving, can actually pull some nutrients out of the bloodstream.

Unfortunately, standard multivitamin-and-mineral pills are not a good way to ensure that your nutritional needs are being met. First, they often don't supply enough of the nutrients needed by the person with CKD. Even worse, they often provide nutrients that you not only don't require but that you shouldn't take. For instance, many contain potassium, phosphorus, or vitamin A, all of which can build up in the blood when kidney function is impaired.

If your blood work shows that you're low in specific nutrients, like vitamin D (see page 48), your doctor will prescribe a supplement for you. Your doctor may also prescribe *renal vitamins*, sometimes referred to as *kidney vitamins*, which are specially formulated to contain the essential nutrients needed by the CKD patient while avoiding phosphorus, potassium, and other nutrients that kidney patients usually *don't* need.

It's important to speak to your doctor about your vitamin and mineral status. If you are already taking a multivitamin, be sure to review the formula with your doctor or dietitian to see if it should be discontinued.

Finally, you'll want to steer clear of certain popular beverages, such as soda, that can be harmful to the individual with chronic kidney disease. (See the inset on page 54.)

FACTORS THAT CAN INFLUENCE OVERALL NUTRITION

As you have learned, the careful selection of foods is essential to keeping your diet as kidney-friendly as possible. However, it's important to keep in mind that various factors—including medications, other health disorders, cultural practices, and more—can also influence your nutritional status. Just as it's vital to understand your dietary needs and restrictions, it's essential to be aware of these additional issues and, as necessary, to discuss them with your doctor or renal dietitian.

Medications

It is not unusual for people with chronic kidney disease to take multiple medications, including prescription medications, over-the-counter products, and natural preparations. Unfortunately, the medications you take can have a great impact on your dietary balance. For instance, some medications, such as certain drugs taken for heartburn, contain sodium. Still other medications can cause stomach upset, reduce your appetite, or cause you to crave foods that aren't good choices, such as salted crackers or sweets.

To make sure that the medications you take interfere with your appetite and mineral balance as little as possible, first, make a complete list of the products you take, including prescribed drugs, over-the-counter preparations, and supplements. (To learn more about supplements and CKD, see the inset on page 52 and the discussion on page 93 of Chapter 5.) Then review this list with your doctor to make sure that the medications are appropriate and the combination doesn't have the potential to do harm. Remember that even "natural" products should be mentioned to your healthcare team, as some of them can have unwanted consequences for the person with CKD. Be sure to read package inserts, too, so that you're aware of possible side effects. And if you find that your appetite is poor, that your stomach is upset, or that you're having unusual cravings, make it a point to tell your doctor, who may be able to adjust your treatment so that you feel better.

Concurrent Medical Conditions

As you have read, CKD can go hand-in-hand with other medical situations that may have an impact on your nutritional status. For example, people with diabetes sometimes develop a digestive problem that causes food to remain in the stomach for an abnormally long period of time. Anemia, which was discussed on page 14, can

---

What Beverages Should Be Avoided When You Have CKD?

As discussed on page 51, when you have CKD, the best beverage is high-quality water, although green tea and fresh fruit and vegetable juices are also good options as long as you choose produce with your dietary restrictions in mind. What about other popular beverages? They can pose problems. First, many of these drinks are high in calories, which can make it harder for you to maintain a healthy weight. Other problems linked to specific beverages are discussed below.

Soda. Soda is not a healthy beverage for anyone, but should be especially avoided by people with chronic kidney disease. The sugar present in non-diet sodas is not only devoid of nutrients but also can result in elevated blood sugar levels, which is harmful for anyone who has diabetes or is at risk for this kidney disease-related disorder. Even diet soda has been linked to diabetes. The high fructose corn syrup used as a sweetener in soft drinks can be even worse than sugar, as it may increase protein leakage into urine by damaging kidney tubules, cause gout and kidney stones, and increase the risk for CKD. Most sodas—especially colas—also contain phosphoric acid, which can cause calcium to leach out of the bones. Finally, many offer a sizeable dose of caffeine, which can decrease calcium absorption and cause bone loss.

result in appetite changes and soreness in the mouth, both of which can cause food to lose its appeal. Additionally, later-stage kidney disease brings an increased risk of depression and acute illness, which can markedly suppress the appetite. And medical conditions like diabetes, heart disease, and hypertension can mean further dietary restrictions.

When you meet with your healthcare team—and especially your dietitian—make sure that everyone is aware of *all* of your health conditions so that your food plan will accurately reflect your nutritional needs. Keep your team up-to-date on new appetite changes or digestive problems so that adjustments can be made in your diet as necessary.

Fruit Juices. Most commercial fruit juice is high in sugar, which, as just discussed, increases the risk of diabetes. Some popular choices also contain too much of the mineral potassium. If you love juices, make them yourself so that you know what's in them, and steer clear of orange, prune, and tomato juice, which are especially high in potassium. Also be sure to practice portion control.

Flavored and Vitamin-Enriched Water. Flavored waters can contain a substance called ChromeMate, which is marketed as a nutrient that balances the body's sugar levels, but is a form of chromium—a mineral that can be toxic if it builds up in the body. In addition, caffeine, added vitamins, artificial flavorings, and sugar or artificial sweeteners—all of which can be a problem for someone with CKD—can be found in some flavored waters. Vitamin waters are usually high in sugar and have added vitamins and minerals that can place a burden on kidneys.

Sports and Energy Drinks. Most sports beverages contain potassium, sodium, phosphorus, and magnesium, which have to be carefully balanced when kidney disease is present. Energy drinks often contain vitamins and herbal products, which can be problematic, as well. Energy drinks also have a high caffeine content, which can lead to bone loss and high blood pressure, and the drinks' high sugar content tends to rapidly increase blood sugar levels.

Cultural and Dietary Preferences

Sometimes, cultural and religious factors have an impact on the CKD patient's ability or desire to follow the recommended renal diet. For instance, your religion may prescribe fasting days or certain dietary prohibitions, or a religious or cultural event may involve certain traditional foods that are at odds with your doctor-prescribed food plan.

First, realize that the consequences may be great if you stray substantially from your diet, and it's wise to make your health a priority. If traditional foods mean a great deal to you, limit the portion size and adjust your daily diet to allow for any components that may be a problem, or, if possible, create a new kidney-friendly version of traditional fare. If it is important to you to eliminate animal products from your diet, you'll be glad to know that vegetarian and vegan diets can be modified to suit the needs of the person with CKD. (See page 74.) Finally, if the renal diet presented to you by your healthcare team conflicts with your cultural or dietary preferences, don't hesitate to discuss the matter with your dietitian so that you can work together to come up with a plan that better meets your needs.

Uremic Symptoms

When kidney disease progresses beyond the early stages, it can result in uremia—a toxic buildup of waste products that can cause a variety of symptoms, including nausea, loss of appetite, and altered taste perception. Clearly, these symptoms can cause you to eat less or choose foods that are less nutritious. Moreover, the weakness, dizziness, or fatigue that can accompany uremia can undermine your intent to shop for and prepare nutritious meals.

Uremia is a serious condition, but it can be treated. If you find yourself experiencing the symptoms just discussed, contact your doctor immediately.

Dialysis

Dialysis changes your dietary needs, because while the process is filtering out toxins and excess fluids from the body, it also removes important nutrients and proteins. Moreover, almost 80 percent of CDK patients undergoing regular dialysis experience gastrointestinal distress due to disorders of both the upper and lower gastrointestinal tract. These problems can, of course, make you feel unwell and reduce your appetite. Similarly, the buildup of wastes that can occur between treatment sessions can make you lose interest in eating.

If you progress to end-stage renal failure and dialysis, your healthcare team will create a special diet that will ensure that you get the nutrients you need, limit the waste products that make you feel unwell, and help you cope with a suppressed appetite. You'll find more about the dialysis diet on page 76 of Chapter 4.

THINGS TO CONSIDER WHEN DINING OUT

So far, this chapter has assumed that you or someone close to you is taking care of both your food shopping and your food preparation, and that you therefore can create the best meals for your dietary needs. But the truth is that most people eat at least some of their meals in restaurants or at other people's homes. In fact, in today's busy world, dining out can be a necessity and not just a social pastime. When CKD is present, eating away from home has the potential to upset the nutrient and fluid levels that you strive to keep in balance. After all, you can't be sure of all the ingredients being used or of the food preparation techniques. Moreover, the available choices may be nothing like the dishes you're accustomed to eating at home, making it hard to select the best foods. Fortunately, there are steps you can take to mirror your recommended diet when dining out.

Eating meals at a friend's or relative's home presents the smallest obstacle to eating kidney-friendly foods. In some cases, you may be comfortable asking your hosts what they're planning to serve and requesting that a portion be prepared to suit your diet—say, with herbs and fresh lemon juice instead of salt. If the meal as a whole is something you shouldn't have, or you feel uncomfortable asking your hosts to make a special meal for you, simply bring a kidney-friendly dish to the get-together. Another option is to eat the food that your hosts provide but to limit the portions with the goal of reducing your intake of problematic nutrients.

Eating at a full-service restaurant presents more of a challenge. Most eateries are increasingly aware of the desire for healthy food choices, and some devote a section of their menu to dishes that are lower in calories and fat. However, the dietary needs of CKD call for great attention to detail regarding ingredients and food preparation. Fast food restaurants are an even bigger test of dietary restrictions, with many venues featuring fried, pre-salted, heavily sauced foods that do not suit your needs at all. When a fast food meal is necessary, however, it's good to know that many fast food restaurants have added grilled or broiled alternatives to their menus and also post the calorie content of every item.

When choosing restaurants, it is advisable to select locations that prepare fresh food to order rather than serving meals from precooked supplies. If you aren't sure about an establishment's cooking policies, inquire ahead of time. Of course, it is wise to restrict your dining to restaurants whose premises appear spotlessly clean. While this practice can't guarantee a sanitary kitchen, clean surroundings can be a good indicator of an emphasis on hygiene. It is also important to be frank with your server about your dietary needs. He or she should know exactly how each menu item is prepared and can either note your special cooking requests or suggest available choices that fit your diet. Lastly, by adopting certain ordering practices, you can make it easier to stick to your recommended diet when dining out. The suggestions below are suitable for almost any restaurant.

❑ Order a small portion. Ask for a child-size, lunch-size, or half-size meal, or share a meal with someone else at the table. This will automatically reduce calories, sodium, potassium, and phosphorus.

❑ Choose a lean meat, and ask that the item be grilled or baked rather than fried.

❑ Substitute extra vegetables for a potato or meat dish.

❑ To limit sodium, request that less cheese or no cheese be used in your meal. Also ask the restaurant to omit bacon and high-sodium and high-fat condiments (such as soy sauce) and seasoning blends. Naturally, you should always request that no salt be added.

❏ Ask that your food be cooked in olive or vegetable oil, rather than butter or margarine. Although it's okay to occasionally use a small amount of butter (less than a teaspoon per serving) in your own cooking, restaurants tend to be lavish in their use of fats, so ask them to substitute oil and to use it sparingly.

❏ Request that sauces and gravies be served on the side or omitted altogether.

❏ Ask that your salad be made of fresh iceberg or romaine lettuce instead of dark green leafy vegetables, and request garnishes of green peppers and cucumber rather than tomatoes, broccoli, or olives. Order low-fat dressing on the side, and ask that cheese and croutons be omitted.

❏ Select water, sparkling water, or sodium-free seltzer over soda, fruit juice, or an alcoholic beverage. Ask for a wedge of lemon or lime to flavor the water or seltzer.

❏ Order a small portion of fruit, sherbet, or sorbet if you are having dessert.

❏ Order coffee black or with nondairy creamer.

Dining out should always be enjoyable. While CKD may bring special dietary considerations, it isn't too difficult to assess menu choices and select the foods and beverages that are the best for your health. By putting your nutritional knowledge to work, doing some advance planning, and sharing your dietary needs with your host or server, you should be able to enjoy meals away from home and still receive the benefits of kidney-friendly eating.

IN CONCLUSION

Protecting your kidney function through diet is a big undertaking but is vital to your well-being. This chapter has presented information about nutrients that bear watching when kidney disease is present, as well as some of the best and worst foods for your renal diet. You have also read about the need to select good-quality food and keep it free of contaminants—which is important to everyone, but is especially necessary to someone with CKD—and you've learned about some of the factors that can affect your nutritional status. You even know strategies that will allow you to dine out without straying from your diet.

Of course, not everyone with CKD has the same nutritional needs. The best diet for you will depend on your stage of CKD; whether you are on dialysis or have had a transplant; any other health disorders you have; and your personal preferences, such as the desire to avoid animal foods. Chapter 4 reviews the various diets that your doctor might recommend based on your health status and presents tips for successfully following each meal plan.

4

Diets Used to Manage CKD

Chronic kidney disease can be diagnosed at different stages and progress in different ways. It can also be accompanied by other health problems—such as hypertension, diabetes, or heart disease—which, like CKD, may involve their own dietary restrictions. It's not surprising, then, that no single dietary plan is right for every person with a kidney disorder.

When considering diets for kidney disease, it's important to understand, too, that nutritional needs can change over time. In the early stages of CKD, there may be no or few restrictions of nutrients because your body may still be able to adequately filter excess chemicals from your blood. As lab work shows that the kidneys have become less able to filter out minerals like potassium and phosphorus, more dietary restrictions may become necessary. But the progression of CKD doesn't necessarily mean that more and more foods will be removed from the menu over time. Under certain circumstances, foods that were formerly restricted may actually reappear on your recommended diet. For instance, even though phosphorus may have previously been restricted on your diet, if new blood tests show low phosphorus levels, your doctor may recommend a diet that provides more of this mineral. If you begin dialysis treatments, the dialysis will eliminate some dietary protein from your body before it can be utilized, requiring you to consume a higher-protein diet. That's why multiple diets, and variations within diets, often come into play in the management of kidney disease.

The diets described below are those most commonly prescribed for people with CKD. In each of the following discussions, you'll learn about the purpose of the diet, discover the foods that are included in it, and find guidance for using the diet successfully to manage your health. Just keep in mind that your own diet—which will be determined by your healthcare team—will be unique and ever-changing.

THE DASH DIET

DASH, an acronym for Dietary Approaches to Stop Hypertension, was originally designed to help people prevent or treat hypertension and has been shown to lower blood pressure within a few weeks. This diet has also been proven to slow the progression of early-stage CKD, making it a good option for people in Stages 1 and 2. (It is higher in potassium, protein, and phosphorus content than is recommended for people in later stages of kidney disease.) In fact, DASH is known to be a lifelong approach to healthy eating for all and is endorsed by doctors, government agencies, the National Kidney Foundation, and the American Heart Association. Studies have shown that it can help with weight control and that it reduces the risk of kidney stones, diabetes, heart disease, stroke, and certain cancers. Moreover, the DASH eating plan is filling, allows for flexibility in food preferences, and can be followed by people of any age.

The DASH diet was created to be low in sodium, high in fiber, low to moderate in fat, and rich in protein, and to offer several key minerals associated with lower blood pressure. It highlights fruits, vegetables, low-fat dairy products, whole grains, poultry, fish, beans, seeds, and nuts, and limits added sugars and sweets, red meats, and fats.

Two forms of this food plan are available—the standard DASH diet, which meets government recommendations of 2,300 mg of sodium per day, and a lower-sodium version, which matches the American Heart Association's daily recommendation of 1,500 mg of sodium. Your age, health, and ethnic background can make a difference in the amount of sodium you should consume.

Below, you'll find the basics of the DASH food plan for about a 2,000-calorie diet. Several websites offer information on following DASH, including tips and sample meal plans. Visit the National Kidney Foundation website for further details. (See page 189.)

❑ Two to two and a half cups a day of fresh fruit.

❑ Two to two and a half cups a day of fresh vegetables.

❑ Six to eight ounces a day of whole grains, such as oatmeal, bulgur wheat, quinoa, or dry cereal (1 ounce equals about $\frac{1}{2}$ cup cooked grains or $1\frac{1}{4}$ cups dry cereal).

❑ Two to three cups a day of low-fat or nonfat dairy products, such as fat-free milk and low-fat yogurt.

❑ Six or fewer ounces a day of lean meats, poultry, or fish.

❑ Four to five days a week, $\frac{1}{3}$ cup nuts, $\frac{1}{2}$ cup cooked legumes (dried beans or peas), 2 tablespoons peanut butter, or 2 tablespoons ($\frac{1}{2}$ ounce) seeds.

❑ Two to three teaspoons a day of fats and oils.

❑ Five tablespoons or less a week of added sugars and sweets such as sorbet and flavored gelatin.

As already mentioned, the DASH eating plan is flexible. Based on your own calorie needs and your blood work, your dietitian can help you shape this diet to better fit your health needs.

DIETS FOR HEART HEALTH

Chronic kidney disease and cardiovascular disease (CVD) are intimately linked, with the development of one disease greatly increasing the odds of getting the other. In fact, the major risk factor for death in kidney patients is heart disease. For this reason, it is not unusual for individuals with CKD to have to blend kidney-friendly eating with a heart-healthy diet.

As you know, a diet for chronic kidney disease involves adjusting your intake of nutrients, minerals, and fluids based on the results of regular blood and urine testing. A heart-healthy diet, on the other hand, mostly focuses on avoiding the consumption of unhealthy fats; increasing the intake of omega-3 fatty acids and fish oil to reduce inflammation; and eating additional fruits, vegetables, and high-fiber foods. (The DASH diet, discussed above, is an excellent eating plan for your heart.) Both kidney and heart-healthy diets have undeniable benefits, but since they have different goals and some discrepancies in the foods they recommend, it's important to confer with both your nephrologist and your cardiologist about the best foods for your personal health.

Let's first look at what heart-healthy and kidney-healthy diets have in common.

❑ Reducing your intake of sodium is good for both your kidneys and your heart. You can help minimize dietary sodium by avoiding fast foods, processed foods, and cured meats, and by avoiding the use of salt when cooking and dining. (For more about sodium, see page 41.)

❑ Decreasing the phosphorus in your diet is also important to both kidney and heart health. Several studies have indicated that higher intakes of phosphorus are associated with an increased risk of cardiovascular disease, and, as you know, phosphorus can build up to unhealthy blood levels when the kidneys are no longer able to filter out adequate amounts. You can control your intake of phosphorus by limiting dairy products and steering clear of packaged, processed, and fast foods. (For more about phosphorus, see page 43.)

❑ Lowering cholesterol through diet and/or medication is a vital part of the management of both heart disease and CKD. You can help reduce your cholesterol intake by avoiding the saturated fats found in full-fat dairy products and red meats, and avoiding the trans fats found in many margarines and commercial baked goods and snacks. (For more about controlling dietary fat, see page 65.)

❑ Reducing protein consumption is important to those people with CKD who are not on dialysis. (Dialysis can pull protein out of your blood, increasing your need for this nutrient.) Limiting animal proteins will also help your heart by decreasing the saturated fat in your diet.

As you can see, many aspects of kidney-friendly and heart-healthy eating mesh very well. However, there are a few areas of conflict:

❑ Limiting sugars and fats is a big part of a heart-healthy diet, yet some people with CKD may need to consume extra carbohydrates and fats to achieve daily calorie goals.

❑ Restricting potassium and phosphorus is important in the management of CKD. But potassium and/or phosphorus are plentiful in many of the vegetables, fruits, nuts, and low-fat dairy products that are part of a heart-healthy diet.

❑ People with heart disease sometimes keep their sodium intake low by using salt substitutes. But many salt substitutes replace sodium chloride with potassium chloride, making this product a bad choice for people with CKD who must limit their potassium consumption.

One factor that we've already touched upon, but is so important that it deserves to be highlighted, is the need to reduce the consumption of the dietary fats that produce lipids in the body. The most significant lipids are cholesterol and triglycerides. *Cholesterol* is necessary for building and maintaining vital parts of your cells, like the cell membranes, and for making bile acids, hormones, vitamin D, and other essential chemicals. This lipid comes in two forms. *Low-density lipoprotein (LDL) cholesterol*, often called "bad" cholesterol, is the main lipid that carries fatty cholesterol to the body tissues. *High-density lipoprotein (HDL) cholesterol*, often referred to as "good" cholesterol, carries excess cholesterol away from your tissues to the liver for removal. *Triglycerides*, another lipid, provide much of the energy needed for your body to function.

While lipids are necessary for life, you can have too much of a good thing. Your doctor will determine if a lower lipid diet is right for you after doing a *lipid panel,* a blood test that measures your cholesterol and triglycerides. A satisfactory blood test shows low LDLs, high HDLs, and low triglycerides, while higher LDLs and triglycerides indicate an increased risk of cardiovascular disease, as well as many other health conditions. At the recommendation of your doctor, you can protect your cardiovascular system by decreasing your intake of dietary fats. The following guidelines should help:

❑ As much as possible, avoid processed and refined foods, which tend to be high not only in fat, but also in salt, potassium, phosphorus, and other substances that you may have to limit.

❑ When you do choose to buy packaged foods, read the Nutrition Facts labels and ingredient lists for information about each item's fat content, and purchase only those foods that will work in your diet. (See the inset on page 36 to learn how to read a food label.) Be aware that the terms "low fat" or "fat free" do not necessarily mean that a product is healthy. The food may actually be high in calories or contain added sugar and sodium.

❑ Avoid packaged foods that contain partially hydrogenated oils. Found mostly in commercial baked goods and in some margarines, this is a form of trans fat, which has been shown to raise bad cholesterol while lowering good cholesterol. Be aware that foods which contain less than .5 gram of trans fat per serving can claim "0 grams of trans fat" in their Nutrition Facts. That's why it's so important to check the ingredients list for partially hydrogenated oils.

❑ Avoid foods prepared with palm or coconut oil, lard, butter, shortening, egg yolks, or whole-milk solids.

❑ Eat oatmeal for breakfast. Oatmeal is known to help reduce blood cholesterol.

❑ Use non-fat milk and dairy products rather than whole milk products.

❑ Use egg whites or cholesterol-free egg substitutes rather than whole eggs.

❑ Aim for five servings a day of fresh fruits and vegetables, and be sure to include grains in your daily diet, selecting only those foods that are a good fit with any restrictions you may have on potassium or other minerals.

❑ Avoid red meat, choosing lean poultry or fish instead. When preparing these foods, remove the fat and skin. Then bake, broil, or roast the meat rather than frying.

❑ To make recipes more heart-friendly, cut the amount of fat by a third or even a half.

❑ When cooking foods, use olive, canola, or soybean oil rather than butter or margarine.

❑ Make your salad dressing with a heart-healthy oil such as extra virgin olive, or avoid the oil entirely and dress your salad with lemon juice or the vinegar of your choice and a sprinkling of herbs.

❑ Flavor your foods with onion, garlic, herbs, and spices instead of butter and other fatty ingredients.

❑ Prepare soups and stews a day ahead, refrigerate overnight, and skim off the fat before reheating.

There is no doubt that following a heart-healthy diet is challenging, especially when it's paired with a diet for kidney health. Your doctor and dietitian will help you create a personalized plan that will accommodate both disorders and improve your overall well-being.

DIETS FOR DIABETES

As you read in Chapter 2, the incidence of diabetes is on the rise. Moreover, while many people with diabetes do not develop CKD, diabetes is the most common cause of kidney problems. With or without kidney disease, people with diabetes need to tightly control the amount of glucose (sugar) in their blood to avoid short- and long-term health problems. For those with CKD, the dangers of poorly controlled blood sugar are even more significant because high levels of glucose cause damage to the filtering units of the kidneys.

There is no single "diabetes diet," since every instance of the condition is unique. Instead, the phrase *medical nutrition therapy* (MNT) is used. MNT is an individualized nutrient-rich, low-fat, low-calorie eating plan that involves consuming moderate amounts of nutritious foods at regularly spaced mealtimes. As you might expect, the type and amount of carbohydrates taken in are particularly important for people with diabetes, because the digestive system breaks this nutrient down into sugar, which the person with diabetes is unable to use properly. There are three ways to manage your carbohydrate intake:

Carbohydrate counting. Carbohydrate counting, or carb counting, helps you keep track of how much carbohydrate you're eating. A limit is set for the amount of carbohydrates you can eat at each meal to help keep blood glucose levels within your target range. You then use food lists and product food labels to track the grams of carbohydrate you consume. Your healthcare team will teach you how to count carbohydrates and, if you take insulin, when to take your insulin and how to adjust the dose.

The glycemic index. You can also choose foods using the glycemic index (GI), a measure of how carbohydrate-containing foods affect blood glucose levels. Items with a high GI raise blood glucose more than foods with a low or medium GI. As you might imagine, low- and medium-GI foods are best for you, although an occasional meal that includes a high-GI food can be balanced by low-GI selections. Your nutritionist or dietitian can teach you more about using the glycemic index to plan your meals.

The exchange system. This plan groups foods into categories, with the foods in each group having a similar amount of carbohydrates per serving. The exchange system allows you to "trade" foods—say, switching one apple for a third cup of pasta—when planning your meal, adding flexibility to your food choices and simplifying the process of tracking carbohydrates.

Just as there are similarities between eating for CKD and eating for heart health, diets for diabetes have factors in common with kidney diets. Here are two similarities:

❏ Reducing your sodium is good for both your kidneys and for diabetes control. (See page 41 for more about limiting sodium.)

❏ Both people with CKD and those with diabetes should avoid cholesterol, saturated fats, and trans fats. So be sure to eliminate or limit red meat, butter, and other sources of saturated fat, and steer clear of margarines, baked goods, and snacks made with trans fats. (See page 66 for more tips on limiting dietary fat.)

There are also several differences between kidney-healthy and diabetes diets:

❏ High-fiber foods are a great way to control diabetes, as they slow the release of glucose into your blood. But some high-fiber foods—such as produce that's high in potassium, or whole grains, which are high in both potassium and phosphorus—often have to be limited or avoided by people with CKD.

❏ People with diabetes are often told to increase their consumption of protein, which slows the release of glucose into the blood. But individuals with chronic kidney disease often must limit their consumption of protein, as protein places stress on the kidneys. (Individuals on dialysis often need *extra* protein.)

❏ It is generally recommended that people with diabetes limit their carbohydrate intake, as too many carbs can elevate blood sugar levels. However, some people with CKD have to consume extra carbohydrates in order to meet their daily calorie goals.

It often seems that the diabetes and kidney diets don't fit well together, but it's important to remember that the control of blood sugar is vital to the control of chronic kidney disease. Your dietitian will work with you to devise an eating plan that will help keep your blood glucose in check while protecting your kidney function.

LOW-PROTEIN DIETS

As you have read, many people with advancing CKD are advised to limit the protein in their diets. Low-protein consumption decreases the production of certain waste products, reduces the workload of the kidneys, and slows the progression of kidney disease. A low-protein diet can also lessen uremic symptoms such as itching and fatigue and has been shown to delay the need for dialysis in people whose CKD has reached Stage 4 or 5. If your blood work shows that there is too much protein in your urine, your doctor may recommend a low-protein diet.

The exact amount of protein recommended for someone on a low-protein diet depends on body weight, nutritional status, CKD stage, and the presence of other medical conditions. Your healthcare team will recommend a daily protein goal and give suggestions for staying within your limits.

Usually, people on a low-protein diet are advised to get half of their daily protein from animal sources like lean poultry and fish. Because these sources are protein-dense, limiting meat portion sizes is important. Each serving should be approximately 3 ounces—about the size of the palm of your hand or a deck of playing cards.

The second half of your daily protein needs should be satisfied by plant sources—vegetables, grains, and legumes (beans, lentils, and peas), for instance. These foods can be consumed in greater quantities than meat without exceeding protein limits. In fact, when you're on a low-protein diet, it is often a good idea to consider vegetables and grains to be the main part of your meals, with a small serving of meat acting as a side dish. For instance, your doctor and renal dietitian may recommend tofu, portobello mushrooms, or lentils as a main dish. Naturally, you should keep any other dietary restrictions in mind as you choose the best plant sources to fill your protein needs. Remember that some of the best plant protein sources are also high in potassium, phosphorus, or both, and these minerals must be limited in the diets of many people with compromised kidneys.

The following guidelines should prove helpful as you follow your low-protein diet:

❑ Be conscientious about staying within your protein limits, but never completely eliminate protein from your diet. This nutrient is required for important body functions such as muscle repair.

❑ To limit protein but still get the nutrients you need, center each meal on vegetables, grains, and other plant sources, and treat meat as a side dish. Chef salads composed mostly of vegetables with small strips of meat or hard-boiled eggs; kebabs made with more vegetables and fruits and smaller pieces of meat; casseroles prepared with more pasta or grains and less meat; and sandwiches that pair small portions of thinly sliced meat with lots of lettuce, cucumbers, and apples are other good ways to lower your protein and still enjoy a nutrient-rich meal.

❑ Allow yourself extra portions or larger servings of bread, rice, and pasta to help meet your caloric needs and to make your meals more filling despite the smaller servings of meat, poultry, and fish. Also consider using more flavorful breads, such as sourdough or rye, and slicing the bread thicker.

❑ When making cream soups, use your favorite milk substitute instead of dairy milk.

❑ Ask your dietitian if you can increase your daily limit of dietary fats. To satisfy your caloric needs, you may be able to use greater amounts of heart-healthy fats such as olive oil and canola oil to cook or season foods.

As always, your healthcare team is the best source of advice regarding your individual dietary needs, and your team will guide you in selecting the best protein sources and portion sizes. Remember that you must also follow any other dietary restrictions your doctor has advised, such as limits on the consumption of potassium, phosphorus, sodium, and/or fluids.

DIETS TO REDUCE KIDNEY STONES

People with chronic kidney disease are at an increased risk of developing kidney stones due to a number of factors, including common problems like polycystic disease and the use of certain medications. For this reason, some people with CKD have to choose foods that reduce the chance that these stones will occur.

Kidney stones develop when chemicals such as calcium, phosphorus, and oxalate (a compound found in many foods) become concentrated and form crystals that accumulate in the urinary system. There are four major types of stones. Calcium stones, especially calcium oxalate stones, are the most common. Following this are uric acid stones; struvite stones, which result from kidney infections; and cystine stones, which are caused by a genetic disorder.

Kidney stones often go unnoticed, but if they move down the urinary tract, they can result in intense pain and bleeding. The recurrent infections and high blood pressure associated with kidney stones can cause CKD to become worse.

Diet is a major factor in kidney stone formation. Individuals who consume a diet high in animal protein, sodium, sucrose (table sugar), and high-oxalate foods are shown to be at greatest risk. A diet that is high in fat and calories may also increase the risk of kidney stones, as can insufficient water intake and inadequate potassium consumption. The DASH diet (see page 62), which limits both animal protein and dietary sodium, is sometimes recommended to help decrease stone formation. Vegetarian diets, which contain little or no animal protein, are also helpful in the avoidance of kidney stones. It is also wise to limit high-oxalate foods, which you'll find listed in the inset on page 73.

Specific dietary guidelines have been shown to help lessen or prevent the formation of kidney stones. While these strategies, shown below, are generally helpful, your ongoing need to balance your intake of minerals and other substances, including fluids, makes it imperative to consult with your healthcare team before making any dietary changes:

❑ Drink enough fluid to maintain a daily urine output of 2 liters (quarts) or more. This may involve drinking nearly 80 ounces of water daily. (To gauge the amount of water that's right for you, measure your urine output for one day.) Increased hydration can significantly reduce the recurrence of stones.

Foods That Can Affect the Risk of Calcium Oxalate Stones

If you have a tendency to get calcium oxalate stones, which are the most common form of kidney stones, your doctor may recommend that you prevent additional stone formation by avoiding foods that have high oxalate levels. The most common high-oxalate foods appear on the list below. Following this list, you'll find one of low-oxalate foods that should *not* increase your risk of oxalate stones. Before changing your diet, either by eliminating foods or by adding new ones, be sure to consult your healthcare team. And remember that when choosing foods for kidney stone prevention, your other dietary restrictions should be kept in mind, as well.

High-Oxalate Foods

Beets	Eggplant	Soy products, such as tofu
Berries	Figs	
Black pepper	Marmalade	Spinach
Celery	Nuts	Swiss chard
Chocolate	Parsley	Tangerines
Cocoa	Peanut butter	Tea (black)
Collards	Purple grapes	Wheat bran
Dark beer	Rhubarb	

Low-Oxalate Foods

Apples and apple juice	Fish (except sardines)	Pork
Cabbage	Green tea	Turkey
Cauliflower	Lemonade	Vegetable oil, all types
Cereals (corn or rice)	Limeade	White bread
Cherries	Milk (low- or no-fat)	White rice
Chicken	Peas	Yogurt (low- or no-fat)
Coffee		

❏ Steer clear of high-oxalate foods. (See the inset on page 73.)

❏ Consume a moderate amount of calcium-rich foods every day, which will reduce the amount of oxalate being absorbed by your body.

❏ Strive for five daily servings of fresh fruits and vegetables that aren't high in oxalate and are also in keeping with your other dietary restrictions. This may increase your intake of potassium, so be sure to talk to your doctor before making dietary changes.

❏ Drink fresh sugar-free lemonade, containing 4 ounces of lemon juice, every day. This increases the amount of citrate in the urine, lowering the chance of stone formation.

❏ Avoid taking vitamin C tablets. Unlike the vitamin C found naturally in foods, large quantities of supplemental vitamin C can increase the amount of oxalate in the urine.

❏ Limit your consumption of sucrose (table sugar) and animal proteins, both of which increase the likelihood of stone formation.

❏ Reduce your intake of sodium. Sodium increases the amount of calcium that's excreted into the urine.

❏ Be diligent about taking the medications prescribed by your doctor. The right medicine, plus dietary adjustments, can keep stones from recurring.

As you can see, the presence of kidney stones adds another level to the dietary modifications that are already part of CKD management. Your doctor and dietitian will guide you in adding or subtracting foods to help prevent additional stones.

VEGETARIAN DIETS

A *vegetarian* diet focuses on plant foods—fruits, vegetables, beans, grains, seeds, and nuts—and does not include meat or seafood. Most vegetarians include dairy products and eggs in their diet, but a small percentage of vegetarians, referred to as *vegans*, do not eat any animal products at all, including dairy products, eggs, and honey. These diets can be helpful with weight control and can effectively lower the risk of kidney disease and kidney stones. They have also been shown to lower the risk of high blood pressure, heart disease, and type 2 diabetes.

Because the consumption of high-quality animal protein is eliminated or sharply limited on a vegetarian diet, there was once concern that this eating plan wasn't compatible with the management of CKD. However, it has been shown that the required amount of protein can definitely be provided by vegetarian and vegan meals. The diet should include a variety of high-quality foods, including soybeans and soy products, such as tempeh and tofu; lentils; beans; and flaxseed oil to provide essential amino acids. Because some vegetarian foods, like beans and lentils, are high in potassium yet important to ensure overall nutrition, low-potassium fruits and vegetables may be added to your diet for balance. Like everyone with CKD, vegetarians and vegans have their blood chemicals closely monitored. When necessary, vitamin and mineral supplements and fortified foods are prescribed to improve nutritional status.

Be sure to discuss your diet with your healthcare team, which will oversee your nutritional status and make sure you get the nutrients you need without overloading on substances that will place stress on your kidneys. Generally, vegetarians with CKD are told to follow these guidelines:

❏ Choose the highest-quality plant proteins, such as tofu, lentils, and beans (especially chickpeas, which are relatively low in potassium).

❏ Aim for the protein intake specified by your healthcare team.

❏ Restrict fruits and vegetables to five servings per day to avoid too much potassium.

❏ Steer clear of excess phosphorus by limiting dairy products to one serving daily.

❏ Avoid eating soy cheese and soy yogurt, which are *very* high in potassium. If you drink soy milk, be aware that different brands have different amounts of phosphorus and potassium. Although food manufacturers are not required to list this information on the

Nutrition Facts label, you will very likely be able to find it online or by contacting the manufacturer.

❑ Always follow your doctor's advice about prescribed nutritional supplements.

With your doctor's guidance and carefully considered food choices, you can reap the benefits of a vegetarian diet while effectively meeting the special nutritional requirements of CKD.

DIALYSIS DIETS

The dialysis process removes toxins and excess fluid from the body when your kidneys can no longer do so. Dialysis can take many forms: standard hemodialysis, which is used for a few hours three times a week at a dialysis center; home or nocturnal hemodialysis, which allows for additional filtration time; and peritoneal dialysis, which is performed every day. The procedure your doctor recommends for you will depend on many factors. But regardless of the chosen dialysis regimen, it's important to realize that dialysis doesn't remove as many toxins and fluids from the body as healthy kidneys can, and that wastes accumulate between dialysis treatments. Moreover, dialysis removes some protein from the blood as it screens out wastes. To keep your fluid and blood chemical levels within a safe range and to make sure that you get the protein you need, careful attention must be paid to what you eat.

Many people who go on dialysis are used to following kidney diets, but once this treatment begins, a dialysis diet is advised. In general, the goals of a dialysis diet are to provide enough protein to fulfill your increased needs; to limit your intake of sodium, potassium, phosphorus, and fluid; and to provide foods that curb inflammation, a condition that is associated with long-term dialysis. Every person who receives this therapy has a unique set of nutritional needs. Your personal dialysis diet will depend upon your blood work, weight, and medications; the kind of dialysis you receive; and any other health problems you have. You can count on your healthcare team to work closely with you to create an eating plan that is perfectly suited to your circumstances. Your team will probably share the following guidelines with you.

❏ Increase your protein consumption. Some protein is lost during the dialysis process, and the procedure changes your body's use of amino acids. High-quality protein sources are recommended to provide the amino acids your body needs without producing too much waste. (See page 35 for information on high-quality proteins.)

❏ Restrict your phosphorus and potassium intake. High-protein foods are often high in phosphorus and potassium, so you'll have to consider the total nutrient content of your food selections carefully. Your healthcare team will help you with this task, and you can also use the low-potassium and low-phosphorus foods lists presented on pages 40 and 44.

❏ Reduce your intake of sodium. A dialysis diet places restrictions on sodium to prevent fluid retention and keep blood pressure under control. (For assistance in limiting your sodium intake, refer to the low-sodium foods list on page 42.)

❏ Limit your fluids to avoid fluid retention, high blood pressure, and heart problems. Remember that ices, ice cream, sherbet, sorbet, gelatin desserts, and soups are considered fluids. The water contained in many fruits and vegetables will also count toward your fluid intake. (To learn more about fluid intake, see page 50.)

❏ Eat more foods that fight the chronic inflammation often found in dialysis patients. A good dialysis diet incorporates foods rich in omega-3 fatty acids and antioxidants. Salmon, red grapes, red bell peppers, and green cabbage are just some of the foods that afford protection against inflammation and the many disorders it can worsen or cause. (To learn more about inflammation and diet, see the inset on page 78.)

Your healthcare team may also advise you to eat four or five smaller meals each day to counter a suppressed appetite, to exercise to maintain muscle mass, and to take medications and supplements exactly as directed to ensure adequate nourishment. It is said that nutrition may be the single most important factor in the success of dialysis. By following your doctor's advice and planning your meals with care, you will take crucial steps to feel your best.

Fighting Chronic Inflammation Through Diet

Chronic inflammation is widely seen in long-term dialysis patients, and has been associated with an increased risk for cardiovascular disease and death. When the inflammatory condition persists—rather than "shutting off," as it does in acute inflammation—the immune system slowly and continuously attacks and damages the internal organs. In the last few years, chronic inflammation has been increasingly identified as an underlying cause of many illnesses, including kidney disease, heart disease, diabetes, and cancer.

Although scientists haven't entirely decoded how chronic inflammation begins and works, they have identified some foods that can combat this dangerous condition. For instance, foods that are high in omega-3 fatty acids—the so-called "good fats"—have been found to "dial down" the white blood cells that cause inflammation in the body. Omega-3 fatty acids can be found in certain fish, including sardines and salmon; in soybeans and soybean products; and in flaxseeds, to name just a few good sources.

Also important to the dialysis diet are fruits and vegetables, which are full of anti-inflammatory substances such as magnesium and antioxidants such as beta-carotene, lycopene, and lutein. Produce that is especially high in these healing nutrients includes red grapes, red bell peppers, carrots, and green cabbage.

When choosing foods to fight inflammation, always keep in mind any restrictions you have on your diet. Speak to your dietitian about the best ways to include antioxidants and omega-3 fats in your daily menu.

DIETS AFTER A KIDNEY TRANSPLANT

When circumstances allow, a transplant may be performed to replace failed kidneys with a healthy, functioning organ. While you should feel much better and face fewer dietary restrictions after a kidney transplant, it is still important to eat right to keep your new kidney healthy and functioning well. By controlling the conditions that originally contributed to your CKD, a transplant diet decreases the chances that your new kidney will suffer damage. The diet also provides the high-quality foods you need to feel your best.

Once you have recovered kidney function, your healthcare team will devise a personalized eating plan based on your lab test results and the number of calories you need to gain, lose, or maintain your weight. Your plan will also include foods that are helpful in the management of high blood pressure and any other health conditions you have. This transplant diet will remain in place for as long as your healthcare team feels it is needed, and, as always, it will be subject to modifications along the way. The following advice may be part of your treatment regimen after having a kidney transplant.

❑ Limit foods that are high in fat and sugar. You may notice an increased appetite due to the immunosuppressant medications you are taking and an improved sense of taste. Many people gain excess weight after a kidney transplant, so it's important to aim for the daily calorie goal set by your dietitian. In addition, diabetes is common after kidney transplant due to both the immunosuppressants and weight gain, making it important to avoid table sugar and products that contain added sugar, sucrose, dextrose, or corn syrup.

❑ Follow a low-sodium diet. Since some immunosuppressants cause fluid and sodium retention, a low-sodium diet is even more important after kidney transplant. Avoid cooking with salt, and buy low- or no-salt products when you shop for food. (To learn more about sticking to a low-sodium diet, see page 41.)

❑ Be sure to include low-fat or no-fat milk and dairy products in your diet. These foods can help you maintain the right levels of calcium and phosphorus without providing more fat than your body needs.

❑ Eat adequate amounts of protein. Your body's protein requirements are high in the first months post-transplant. Your doctor and dietitian may ask you to increase your intake of high-quality protein as your body heals from the stress of major surgery. In addition, some transplant medications can cause a breakdown of protein in the body and create the need for more of this nutrient. Lean meats, skinless poultry, fish, lentils, and beans provide high-quality protein without adding excess fat to your diet.

❏ Make sure you get adequate fiber. Follow your dietitian's advice about fiber to help maintain your digestive health. (See page 47 to learn more about fiber.)

❏ Stay sufficiently hydrated by taking in adequate amount of water and other fluids. Your healthcare team will tell you how much fluid is right for your individual needs.

❏ Consume at least five servings of vegetables and fruits daily once

Protecting Against Gout Through Diet

Earlier in this book (see page 12), you learned that while healthy kidneys can filter out and eliminate excess acids, including uric acid, chronic kidney disease allows blood acid levels to rise. One of the health problems associated with high uric acid levels is gout.

Gout occurs when uric acid builds up and forms crystals in the joints, causing pain, swelling, and stiffness, and making it difficult to move. Gout can even cause deformity of the joints. Just as CKD can lead to the development of gout, it is now known that gout can lead to the development and worsening of chronic kidney disease.

Fortunately, smart dietary choices can help keep uric acid levels in check. Eating a diet high in vegetables and fruits is a good first step to avoiding gout, as this will help your body maintain acid-alkaline balance. You'll also want to avoid foods that are particularly high in the naturally occurring chemicals known as purines, as uric acid results from the body's breakdown of these chemicals. On the next page, you'll find a list of foods that are high in purines, and should be avoided, as well as a list of foods that are low in these substances. If you are prone to getting gout, you'll want to talk to your doctor about other ways in which you can lower your risk. And remember that when choosing low-purine foods, you must also keep other dietary restrictions in mind.

you recover kidney function. Your doctor will monitor the phosphorus and potassium in your blood and let you know if restrictions are necessary. As mentioned throughout this book, fresh fruits and vegetables are among the healthiest food choices.

❏ Avoid grapefruit and grapefruit juice. These items contain a substance that can negatively affect the actions of several immunosuppressants. Substitute other fruits and juices.

❏ Practice safe food handling to lower the risk of infection. Immunosuppressant drugs reduce your body's ability to combat disease, so whether dining at home or at a restaurant, you'll want to make cleanliness and food safety a priority. (See the inset on page 32 for information on keeping your food safe.)

High-Purine Foods

Alcohol, especially beer	Mackerel	Sardines
Anchovies	Mushrooms	Scallops
Asparagus	Mussels	Spinach
Cauliflower	Organ meats, such as heart, kidney, liver, and sweetbreads	Yeast
Gravies		
Herring		
High-fat foods		

Low-Purine Foods

Bread (not whole grain)	Eggs	Vegetable oil, all types
Cereals (not whole grain)	Fruits	Vegetables (avoid those high in purines)
Cheese (low-fat or no-fat)	Herbs	
	Popcorn	
Cornbread	Rice (white)	Vinegar

In addition to following your transplant diet, be sure to take medications and supplements exactly as prescribed, and follow your doctor's advice about exercise, alcohol consumption, and other lifestyle choices. (See Chapter 5 for more about these topics.)

IN CONCLUSION

As you have learned in this chapter, the right dietary choices are critical when kidney disease is present. As CKD progresses, the foods you eat will play a major role in protecting your remaining kidney function and enhancing your overall health. Even when renal failure occurs and dialysis or a kidney transplant enters the picture, your diet will have a significant effect on how your body responds and how you feel.

Although this chapter has discussed several different food plans, you have read that each diet must be geared to individual needs and determined by the stage of the kidney disease, any other health conditions, and the results of laboratory tests, which change over time. Sometimes, the most appropriate nutritional plan may be a blend of two different diets. In addition, personal nutrient goals—which may include the restriction of certain foods or the inclusion of particular foods or food combinations—often come into play.

No one knows more about the state of your kidneys than your healthcare team, so the advice of your doctor and dietitian should always be the foundation of your dietary plan. You can help your team and yourself by keeping a diary of the foods you eat, along with the quantities consumed. Reviewing your diary at each office visit will enable your doctor to discuss any risks that may be presented by your food choices. It can also give you extra confidence in the benefits and safety of your kidney diet.

5

$\mathscr{I}$mportant Steps to Maximizing Your Health

Throughout the first four chapters of this book, you learned about kidney function, kidney dysfunction, and the role that diet can play in both causing and managing chronic kidney disease. You now know that to effectively control your kidney problem, it is vital to follow the food plan that your healthcare team provides. But there are many other steps you can take to improve not just your kidney function but also your overall health. The road to maximizing your well-being begins by accepting responsibility for your treatment; learning everything you can about your health condition, including the many resources that are available to you; and working closely with your healthcare team. You can then make some simple lifestyle changes that will enhance both your level of fitness and the overall success of your treatment. This chapter was designed to guide you in doing all you can to enjoy a longer, healthier life.

BECOME AN ACTIVE PARTICIPANT IN YOUR TREATMENT PROGRAM

It's not always easy to accept the diagnosis of chronic kidney disease, but recognizing the problem, learning all you can about it, and becoming actively involved in your treatment program will help you feel better, both physically and emotionally, and even allow you to slow the progression of CKD. While this may sound like a tall order, the following discussions outline the many things you can do to take control of your health.

Learn Everything You Can About Your Health Condition and Its Treatment

While some patients are eager to learn about CKD and understand the many aspects of successful treatment, many others avoid researching the disorder due to a lack of time, low energy, the simple fact that CKD is an unsettling subject, or even because they still feel well. Some people, in fact, refuse to accept their diagnosis and therefore don't take the steps necessary to manage their disease.

If you are having trouble coming to terms with your diagnosis, speak to your healthcare team about getting emotional support. It is not unusual for people to feel overwhelmed by the prospect of coping with CKD. Fortunately, assistance is available in the form of one-to-one therapy, support groups, and online discussion forums that can connect you to patients who are dealing with various stages of chronic kidney disease.

Usually, as people gain knowledge about their condition, they feel calmer and more in control of their lives. This is good news, as the more you know about chronic kidney disease, the better equipped you will be to follow your healthcare team's recommendations and make smart decisions about diet, medication, and other aspects of your treatment plan. This can pay enormous dividends in the form of slower progression of your CKD and better management of any symptoms. Reading this book is a good first step on the road to knowledge. Also ask your doctor and renal dietitian about any handouts they may be able to supply, including pamphlets about CKD, printed dietary guidelines, and recipes that fit your dietary needs and limitations. (Turn to page 97 for a collection of easy-to-follow kidney-friendly recipes.) Just as important, be aware of the many organizations that make information available on this subject. If you turn to the Resources section, which begins on page 183, you'll find contact information for the American Kidney Fund, the National Kidney Foundation, and other groups that offer information on chronic kidney disease and associated disorders; useful tips for making dietary and lifestyle changes; basic facts about dialysis and kidney transplants; advice on weight management; and much more.

Learn About Available Financial Assistance

In addition to the need for information, kidney patients often require financial help. If you are in the early stages of CKD, you may find that the foods recommended on your renal diet are more expensive than the foods you're used to eating. The costs of doctor's visits, laboratory testing, and medications can also add up, and if dialysis or kidney transplant comes into the picture, the costs can be prohibitive if you don't have sufficient insurance.

Once again, your healthcare team can be your best resource. They can arrange for financial counseling, direct you to sources of community or government assistance, and work with you to prevent finances from becoming a factor in your treatment. Also check out the organizations listed in the Resources section. (See page 183.) Several groups, such as the American Kidney Fund, offer financial help to people who need assistance in paying for CKD-related treatment.

Work Actively With Your Healthcare Team

Once you have accepted your diagnosis and are ready to make necessary dietary and lifestyle changes, you'll find that the members of your healthcare team are the best possible sources of information, answers, advice, and support. These professionals will become familiar with your medical history, will continually monitor the state of your health, and will quickly come to know you as a person, as well. Of course, the more actively you work with them, following the program of treatment they provide and giving them candid information about your daily eating choices and the way you feel, the more successful you will be in your efforts to control CKD. The following suggestions can help ensure that your treatment proceeds without a hitch.

❏ Keep all of your office and lab appointments. As you have learned throughout this book, monitoring your lab results and general health is crucial to protecting your kidney function. Only by checking your blood work on a regular basis will your healthcare team be able to fine-tune your diet and adjust your medications as necessary.

❏ Do your best to follow all your doctor's recommendations. There is a great deal involved in CKD management, and it won't always be easy to adhere to all of your treatment team's advice. Remember that doing so is your key to a longer, healthier life.

❏ Be an active member of your healthcare team. Don't hesitate to ask questions about your treatment, to take notes, or to request the clarification of instructions.

❏ Take your medication exactly as prescribed. If taken incorrectly, some medications can cause digestive upset or decreased appetite that may affect your nutritional status.

❏ Be honest about what you are eating. Slip-ups or variations from your recommended diet can alter your lab results. Your healthcare team needs to know if there is a reason for the change in your labs.

❏ Tell the truth about the way you feel, both physically and emotionally. New or troubling symptoms can be a sign that your condition has changed or that you need some help in coping with CKD and its treatment. The professionals on your team are there to support you.

The importance of knowledge, involvement, and compliance during the management of your condition is stressed throughout this chapter. As you can imagine, procrastination, inconsistency, or disregard of professional advice will unintentionally undermine your efforts to preserve the health of your kidneys. Always remember that a positive attitude goes a long way toward helping you feel vital, empowered, and in control of your condition.

MAKE HEALTHY LIFESTYLE CHANGES

You already know the important difference you can make by choosing kidney-friendly foods and avoiding foods that can place a strain on your kidneys. But if you want to truly maximize your health, there is much more you can do to manage CKD and enhance your overall well-being. While some of the following changes may prove challenging, they are sure to provide lasting rewards.

Manage Your Weight

Maintaining proper body weight is essential to CKD management. This is why your weight will be tracked as part of every office visit. Your *body mass index* (*BMI*)—a measure of weight in relation to height—may also be recorded.

Because of dietary limitations and loss of appetite, some people with CKD have trouble keeping their weight sufficiently high. Throughout the course of the disease, it's important to consume enough *calories*—the energy in food that keeps your body running—to prevent unintended weight loss that can sap your energy and signal inadequate nutrition. If you do lose weight unexpectedly, your healthcare team will suggest safe ways to add extra calories to your diet. Kidney-friendly nutritional drinks such as Nepro, Suplena, and Magnacal Renal may be recommended if your team determines that you need nutritional supplementation. Bear in mind that some nutritional drinks may contain excessive amounts of potassium and other minerals, so be sure to talk to your doctor before using any supplemental product.

What if your weight is higher than it should be? Being overweight and carrying too much body fat increases the risk of CKD and also speeds the progression of the condition. Therefore, if you have kidney disease and are carrying extra pounds, your healthcare team will work with you to attain a healthier weight. Losing excess weight may not only slow the decline of kidney function but also decrease the amount of protein in your urine and lower your blood pressure. Simply sticking to the diet advised by your doctor and dietitian will often help you attain a better weight. You may also be asked to track the calorie content of the foods and beverages you consume each day and to exercise more to help your body burn additional calories. The inset found below provides tips on losing weight and keeping it off, and the next discussion will guide you in increasing your level of activity.

Engage in Regular Physical Activity

Exercise can go a long way toward improving your overall health. In fact, many serious diseases have been linked to a combination of poor diet and physical inactivity. It is well known that the best outcomes

---

Weight-Loss Tips

The secret to weight loss is actually very simple: Burn more calories than you eat. Of course, the reality of losing unwanted pounds is not that easy. The following tips can help you work toward and maintain your ideal weight. Just keep in mind that as you choose the foods for your weight-loss diet, you should always consider your other dietary restrictions so that your meals are both weight- and kidney-friendly.

☐ Keep track of your calories. Information about the calorie content of everyday foods is available on food labels, in books, and online. There are many apps available to help you with calorie-counting, or you can keep a food diary that lists everything you eat or drink along with each item's calorie content. On average, a man needs about 2,500 calories daily to maintain his weight while a woman requires around 2,000 calories. Your dietitian can provide calorie guidelines that are specific to your needs.

☐ Cut down on portion sizes. If your normal breakfast is an English muffin (120 calories) with a tablespoon of spreadable fruit (35 calories) and an 8-ounce glass of juice (95 calories), consider eating only half of a muffin and combining 4 ounces of juice with 4 ounces of water. You'll save 125 calories before 9:00 AM—and you'll avoid the excess potassium found in many popular fruit juices.

among people with chronic kidney disease are enjoyed by those who monitor their weight and increase their activity level. This healthy combination can lower both blood pressure and cholesterol, strengthen bones, improve heart rates, enhance mood, and help people enjoy a better quality of life. Although you may have felt tired or ill prior to your diagnosis, the proper management of your condition should soon have you feeling better. At this point, getting daily exercise is one of the most beneficial things you can do for yourself. It's important to consult with your doctor before undertaking any new physical activity. Your treatment team knows your medical history as well as the particulars of your CKD and general health and can offer exercise suggestions that suit you perfectly.

□ Read food labels. The calorie and sugar contents of one serving are clearly listed in an item's Nutrition Facts. You can also learn whether a food has added sugar, which may be listed as sugar, sucrose, dextrose, or fructose. The food label will also tell you about the presence of sodium, saturated fats, and trans fats, all of which can prevent weight loss while compromising kidney health.

□ Avoid sugary foods and sweetened beverages. This includes sodas, juices, cakes, cookies, pastries, ice cream, and candy. Consider eliminating dessert from your meals, and plan ahead so you have appealing low-calorie food choices on hand for snacking.

□ Decrease or eliminate the alcohol in your diet. Beer, wine, and mixed drinks are packed with calories. Try substituting sparkling water on ice with a twist of lemon or lime. (To read more about alcohol and CKD, see page 93.)

□ Set manageable weight-loss goals. It's hard to become motivated to lose forty pounds, but it's easy to set out to lose five. When you've lost the first five pounds, set a new goal of ten, and so forth.

It's important to view your weight-loss diet as a healthy, permanent eating plan. Doing so is good for your health and is the surest way to keep unwanted pounds from creeping back.

Physical activity can take many forms. If you were previously a sedentary person, getting thirty minutes of moderate physical activity each day will be a big change. Examples of moderate exercise include brisk walking, dancing, bicycling, light weight training, yard work, and doubles tennis. If you are reasonably active, increasing your exercise level will mean engaging in more vigorous pursuits such as jumping rope, playing basketball, swimming, or running. Regardless of the form of exercise you add to your daily life, the physical and emotional benefits will be significant. You may initially find it hard to increase your activity level, especially if you are generally inactive or haven't been feeling well. The inset on page 91 offers ideas that will help you get started.

Limit Caffeine and Chocolate

Coffee, tea, cappuccino, lattes, hot chocolate, and soda are popular beverages that often contain caffeine. Many sports and energy drinks also list caffeine among their ingredients. The effect of caffeine on people with kidney disease is not clear, but it is known that the substance can cause a loss of calcium, particularly if you have a low level of vitamin D. In addition, caffeine acts as a diuretic and can interfere with proper hydration. It can also cause a short-term spike in blood pressure. As you know, these properties can be a problem for someone with CKD. It's also important to remember that many of these beverages contain substances—namely, sodium, potassium, and phosphorus—that may be restricted in people with kidney disease. Depending on preparation and sugar content, they may also be very high in calories. It is wise to talk to your healthcare team about the amount of caffeine that is right for you. Often, a two-cup daily limit on coffee and tea is advised. Your doctor and dietitian can recommend other beverages that will help you stay within your caffeine limits.

Recently, the health benefits of dark chocolate have been touted. This food contains many beneficial compounds, including antioxidants, vitamins, minerals, and healthy fats. In fact, it is said that dark chocolate and cocoa can help decrease blood pressure and lipid levels and may also reduce the risk of heart disease. However, chocolate

Simple Ways to Develop the Exercise Habit

There are a number of reasons people give for avoiding physical activity—among them, fatigue, disinterest, and lack of energy or time. When you are dealing with a chronic illness that makes you feel unwell, keeping fit may seem like a gargantuan task. But exercise is much more than a pastime; it's essential to your physical and emotional health. Here are some ideas for adding physical activity to your life.

☐ Set time limits on sedentary activities like watching television or browsing online. Trim fifteen minutes each day from the time you spend sitting still.

☐ Add exercise to your sedentary time. Use a stationary bike or treadmill as you read or watch TV, or pedal a foot cycle or march in place when using your computer.

☐ Start exercising at a gradual pace. Begin with ten to fifteen minutes of activity, and add five minutes every day.

☐ Pick an appealing activity. Dance, swing a golf club at a driving range, or take a walk in a park or at the beach.

☐ Alternate your forms of exercise. Avoid monotony by biking one day and hiking in the woods the next.

☐ Walk with a partner or listen to music as you work out. Conversation and music can be pleasant distractions.

☐ Wear a pedometer and aim to take 10,000 or more steps a day.

☐ Chart your exercise level by keeping a diary of the time and duration of your activities. You'll be proud of this record of your progress.

If you have CKD, regular exercise is an important addition to the management of your condition. By experimenting with the suggestions listed above, you'll find it easier to enjoy the many benefits of increased physical activity.

and cocoa are sources of caffeine as well as potassium and phosphorus. Also, foods made with chocolate usually contain sugar, carbohydrates, saturated fats, and minerals that are limited in kidney diets.

If chocolate is permitted in your kidney diet, it's advisable to eat tiny portions of only dark chocolate, only once in a while. Prepare cocoa using hot water instead of milk, and use two teaspoons of powder rather than the usual four. As always, be sure to talk to your healthcare team before adding anything new to your diet.

Quit Smoking

There is plenty of evidence that smoking is bad for your health. For people with CKD, this habit poses special risks. Smoking has been shown to speed up the progression of kidney disease. The nicotine in tobacco impairs the body's absorption of several vitamins, especially vitamins D and C, and reduces blood flow to the kidneys. Smoking also increases the risk of protein leaking into the urine, as well as that of hypertension and cardiovascular disease, two conditions that often go hand-in-hand with CKD. It is also known to alter the senses of taste and smell, causing smokers to eat foods excessively high in sodium, phosphorus, and potassium. Moreover, it is known that people with diabetes who smoke tend to develop kidney problems earlier and lose kidney function sooner than those who never smoked or have quit smoking. The Centers for Disease Control and Prevention warns that smoking is harmful to every organ in your body. There is no doubt that this habit will undermine your efforts to protect your kidneys.

If you smoke, ideally, you should quit immediately. Your healthcare team can advise you about medications, therapies, and stop-smoking programs that can help you through the process and provide encouragement as you take this very important step. If you do not plan to quit, at the very least, try to decrease the amount you smoke. You can do this by noting the times of day and activities during which you smoke, and changing your routine to avoid the scenarios linked to smoking. Of all the lifestyle changes you can make, this may be the one that offers the greatest benefits for your overall health and the well-being of your delicate kidneys.

Limit Alcohol Use

In healthy adults, minimal alcohol consumption—defined as one drink per day for women and older adults and one to two drinks per day for men—usually causes no problems. In fact, it has been suggested that light alcohol use may actually be good for you. Red wine, in particular, offers antioxidants and other substances that are said to have beneficial effects on HDL levels and heart health. Consuming more than a minimal amount of alcohol can be a problem, however, especially if you have CKD or blood pressure problems. Having more than one to two drinks per day can increase blood pressure, interfere with medications, cause problems with blood sugar and chemical levels, and damage kidney cells, thereby causing CKD to become worse. In addition, regardless of your state of health, heavy alcohol consumption is linked to weight gain, a decline in nutritional status, liver problems, cancer, and cardiovascular disease.

If you do not drink, do not begin after you've learned that you have kidney problems. If you do drink and have CKD, it is imperative that you ask your doctor or dietitian if minimal alcohol consumption is safe for you. Once you have received your doctor's permission to have an occasional alcoholic beverage, be sure to monitor the ingredients and nutrient content of each drink. Many drinks containing alcohol—wine and beer, for instance—also contain sodium, potassium, and phosphorus that can throw off your blood chemical levels. Also, if you have edema or are on dialysis, you must count alcoholic drinks as part of your daily fluid allowance. With your doctor's approval, you can enjoy an occasional drink and still protect your kidneys. Simply be aware of potential risks, and keep your consumption of alcohol to a minimum.

Avoid Nutritional Supplements Unless They Are Prescribed

According to recent studies, well over half of the adults in the United States regularly take supplements, including vitamin-and-mineral products and herbals. Many people view supplementation as part of a healthy lifestyle and use it to "fill in nutrient gaps" in their diets. But are these nutritional supplements right for people with CKD?

Multivitamin-and-mineral pills can be a source of trouble for individuals with chronic kidney disease. Because impaired kidneys cannot control nutrient levels, over-the-counter multivitamins can upset the balance of blood chemicals. It is especially important to avoid taking supplements that contain potassium, phosphorus, and vitamins A, E, C, and K unless instructed to do so by your doctor.

As you learned in Chapter 3, if you are found to be deficient in vitamin D or calcium, your physician may prescribe activated vitamin D and/or calcium supplements. Your healthcare team may also recommend kidney-friendly renal supplements such as ProRenal Vital, ProRenal QD, Renaltab I, Nephrocaps, or Nephro-Vite. If you are now taking a supplement, be sure to let your nephrologist know. Never use any preparation without the approval of your healthcare team.

Because people tend to view herbal products as being "natural," they often assume that they're safe, but some of these substances can do great harm, especially when chronic kidney disease is present. As you may already know, there are tens of thousands of herbal products on the market, and many new items are introduced every year. However, these products are not regulated by the FDA, and some have been found to contain potentially dangerous substances not listed on the label—or to omit the primary ingredient that *is* listed on the label. This means that if you take these products, you may unknowingly consume extra nutrients that are restricted for people with CKD and, perhaps, fail to receive the nutrients you desire.

Even when herbal supplements are properly prepared and contain only the ingredients listed, it's important to understand that they are powerful substances that can have drug-like effects. For example, echinacea, an immune stimulant, and St. John's wort, a mood stabilizer, can interact with anti-rejection medications after a kidney transplant. Other herbs can impede the body's absorption of medications and carefully balanced nutrients. Still other herbal products have been directly linked to the formation of kidney stones and complete kidney failure. The National Kidney Foundation, which cautions against using herbal supplements if you have CKD, states that the following supplements are especially risky for people at any stage of the disease:

Herbs to Avoid

Apium graveolens	Horsetail	Oregon grape root
Astralagus	Huperzinea	Parsley root
Barberry	Java tea leaf	Pennyroyal
Cat's claw	Licorice root	Ruta graveolens
Creatine	Nettle, stinging nettle	Uva ursi
Goldenrod		Yohimbe

As always, the bottom line is that before you use any herbal supplement, you must obtain your doctor's approval so that he or she can consider potential drug interactions and your particular health condition.

IN CONCLUSION

There is so much you can do to feel better, help protect your kidneys, and reduce the chance that you'll be affected by heart disease and other illnesses associated with CKD. Start by learning about chronic kidney disease and getting actively involved in your treatment plan. This will not only give you valuable information about your condition but will also supply the motivation you need to do the hard work of caring for yourself. Then start introducing lifestyle modifications that can make a real difference. When all is said and done, following a kidney diet and adopting a healthful lifestyle are the best actions you can take to treat your CKD.

PART TWO

$\mathscr{K}$idney-Friendly Recipes

In Part One, you learned the basics of kidney function and kidney disease. You also learned about the link between chronic kidney disease and diet, and how smart food choices can be used to reduce the strain on kidneys and enhance your overall health. Still, you may be a little uncertain about how you can put your new knowledge into practice to create tasty kidney-friendly dishes. That's what Part Two is all about. It's a treasure trove of over fifty recipes specially designed for people with CKD.

Created by dietitians, the recipes in the following pages offer a diverse range of dishes, including breakfast treats, entrées, side dishes and salads, sauces and dressings, snacks, and desserts. Each recipe begins by listing the CKD diets with which that dish is generally compatible, as well as the types of diets with which it is generally *not* compatible. In a few cases, the recipe also includes a note about specific nutrients that may be a little high for some people. In creating these dishes, our goal has been to meet the needs and limitations of *most* people with CKD. Remember, though, that everyone's needs are different, so if you're in doubt about the suitability of a dish, you'll want to check it out with your doctor or dietitian before adding it to your meal plan. The Nutritional Facts Per Serving, provided at the end of each recipe, will allow you and your healthcare team to evaluate it with ease, as these facts provide counts for calories, protein, carbohydrates, fiber, fat, saturated fat, trans fat, cholesterol, phosphorus, potassium, and sodium per serving. You'll even find a listing of diabetic exchanges.

When creating menu plans with dietary limitations in mind, be sure to look at the nutrients provided by your *entire meal*, and not just each individual dish. For instance, in addition to your Spicy Chicken Sandwich (page 114), you may also choose to have a portion of Chopped Salad page 135). It's important to add up the *total nutrients* that meal will provide. When looking through the Entrées section (pages 112 through 129), you may find that most dishes—Kung Pao Chicken (page 112) and Steak Fajita Pita (page 118), for instance—are actually complete meals. The nutrient counts may seem a little high per serving, but for most people with CKD, these one-dish meals will not exceed per-meal limits for fat, sodium, potassium, or phosphorus.

In creating the following recipes, we never lost sight of the fact that besides being kidney-friendly, each dish should be easy to prepare and delicious. That's why, from Vegetable Frittata to Old-Fashioned Baked Cinnamon Apples, you'll find straightforward listings of ingredients followed by simple step-by-step directions that help ensure success. These recipes require no special or tricky techniques, nor do they call for hard-to-find ingredients.

As you read the following recipes, you may see that they have certain things in common. Whenever possible, fresh foods have been used rather than processed foods to keep potassium, sodium, and phosphorus at a minimum. The emphasis on fresh ingredients also eliminates unhealthy preservatives and other additives. When canned foods have been used for the sake of convenience, lower-sodium or no-salt-added products have been specified. To reduce cholesterol, whole eggs are often mixed with egg whites or egg replacement; and to keep protein at a healthy level, meat, poultry, and other high-protein foods have been modestly portioned. Cheese has been used only sparingly, just to add flavor and a bit of creaminess; and whenever ingredients are cooked in a skillet, they are sautéed in a small amount of heart-healthy oil rather than butter. You might want to use these principles to revamp your own family recipes so that they can be incorporated in your CKD diet. Just keep in mind that portion control is vital. It's one of the tricks that allows you to eat many of the foods you like without getting more protein, fat, phosphorus, potassium, or sodium than your body can handle.

So choose a recipe, buy some fresh and flavorful ingredients, and get ready to enjoy delicious kidney-friendly dishes.

BREAKFAST DISHES

OVERNIGHT SLOW-COOKER OATS

Check with your doctor or dietitian to make sure that this recipe is compatible with your current dietary needs and limitations.

YIELD: 8 SERVINGS

• • • • • •

8$\frac{1}{2}$ cups water

2 cups uncooked steel-cut oats

1$\frac{3}{4}$ cups rice milk

$\frac{1}{4}$ cup packed brown sugar

1 teaspoon vanilla extract

1. Line the insert of a slow cooker with a plastic slow-cooker liner, and spray the liner with cooking spray.

2. Place all of the ingredients except for the vanilla extract in the slow cooker, and stir to combine.

3. Cover and cook on low for 7 to 8 hours, or until the oats are cooked through and creamy. Stir in the vanilla extract and serve immediately. Leftovers can be stored in individual serving-size containers, frozen, and reheated in the microwave oven.

NUTRITIONAL FACTS PER SERVING			
• • • • • •		Fat	3.5 g
		Sat Fat	0.5 g
		Trans Fat	0 g
Calories	210	Cholesterol	0 mg
Protein	6 g	Phosphorus	21 mg
Carbohydrates	38 g	Potassium	175 mg
Fiber	4 g	Sodium	40 mg

DIABETIC EXCHANGES
• • • • • •
2 starch
.5 other carbs

TROPICAL SMOOTHIE

Check with your doctor or dietitian to make sure that this recipe is compatible with your current dietary needs and limitations.

YIELD: 2 SERVINGS

• • • • • •

8 ounces vanilla soy
   yogurt

$1/2$ large banana, cut
   into chunks

$1/2$ cup chunks fresh
   pineapple

$1/4$ cup passion fruit juice

1. Place all of the ingredients in a blender and process on high speed until thick and smooth.

2. Divide between 2 glasses and serve immediately.

NUTRITIONAL FACTS PER SERVING			
• • • • •		Fat	3 g
		Sat Fat	0 g
		Trans Fat	0 g
Calories	180	Cholesterol	0 mg
Protein	5 g	Phosphorus	18 mg*
Carbohydrates	33 g	Potassium	384 mg*
Fiber	2 g	Sodium	15 mg

DIABETIC EXCHANGES
• • • • • •
1 fruit
.67 milk (skim)
.67 other carbs

* The phosphorus and potassium data presented for this recipe were calculated using one brand of soy yogurt. Because these nutrients can vary from brand to brand, be sure to contact the manufacturer of the yogurt you choose to determine if that brand will meet your nutritional needs.

BAKED OATMEAL WITH BERRIES

Check with your doctor or dietitian to make sure that this recipe is compatible with your current dietary needs and limitations.

YIELD: 4 SERVINGS

• • • • • •

1 large egg

$^1/_3$ cup unsweetened applesauce

$1^1/_2$ tablespoons packed brown sugar

$1^1/_2$ cups uncooked old-fashioned oats (cook in 5 minutes)

$^1/_2$ cup nonfat milk

$^1/_2$ teaspoon double-acting baking powder

$^1/_2$ teaspoon ground cinnamon

$^1/_4$ teaspoon ground allspice

$^1/_4$ teaspoon vanilla extract

$^1/_2$ cup fresh raspberries

1. Preheat the oven to 350°F. Spray an 8 x 8-inch baking dish with cooking spray, and set aside.

2. Place the egg, applesauce, and brown sugar in a large bowl, and stir to mix. Add all of the remaining ingredients except for the raspberries, and stir until mixed and well-moistened.

3. Pour the egg mixture into the prepared pan, and arrange the raspberries over the top.

4. Bake for 25 to 30 minutes, or until the mixture is firm and a knife inserted in the middle comes out clean or has moist crumbs clinging to it.

5. Serve warm, at room temperature, or chilled.

NUTRITIONAL FACTS PER SERVING			
• • • • •			
Calories	180	Fat	3.5 g
Protein	7 g	Sat Fat	.5 g
Carbohydrates	32 g	Trans Fat	0 g
Fiber	4 g	Cholesterol	45 mg
		Phosphorus	199 mg
		Potassium	223 mg
		Sodium	95 mg

DIABETIC EXCHANGES
• • • • • •
1.5 starch
.24 meat (medium fat)
.28 fruit
.12 dairy (skim)
.39 other carbs

FOR:

■ DASH Diet
■ Diabetes Diet
■ Dialysis Diet
■ Heart Health Diet
■ Kidney Stone
   Reduction Diet
■ Low-Protein Diet
■ Post-Transplant Diet
■ Vegetarian Diet

VEGETABLE FRITTATA

Check with your doctor or dietitian to make sure that this recipe is compatible with your current dietary needs and limitations.

YIELD: 3 SERVINGS

• • • • • •

4 ounces sugar snap peas, stems trimmed, cut into $1/2$-inch pieces

2 large eggs

2 large egg whites or $1/3$ cup liquid egg whites

$1/4$ teaspoon ground turmeric

Freshly ground black pepper to taste

$1/3$ cup chopped scallions

$1/4$ cup chopped red bell pepper

2 tablespoons chopped fresh dill, or $1/4$ teaspoon dried dill

1 teaspoon olive or canola oil

$1/4$ cup shredded Parmesan cheese

1. Steam or boil the sugar snap peas for 2 to 3 minutes, or just until tender. Rinse under cold water to stop further cooking, drain, and pat dry.

2. Place the eggs, egg whites, turmeric, and black pepper in a medium-size bowl, and whisk until the mixture is well blended. Stir in the prepared sugar snap peas, scallions, red pepper, and dill. Set aside.

3. Preheat the broiler. Brush the oil over an oven-safe 10-inch nonstick skillet with sloping sides, and heat the skillet over medium-low heat.

4. Pour the egg mixture into the skillet. Cook for 2 to 4 minutes, or until the bottom is lightly browned. During cooking, lift the edges with a spatula and tilt the skillet from time to time so that the uncooked egg flows underneath.

5. Once the egg is set around the edges and starting to firm up in the middle, transfer the skillet to the broiler and cook for 3 to 5 minutes, or until the top is lightly browned and the mixture is firm to the touch. Rotate the skillet as necessary for even browning.

6. Remove the pan from the oven, and sprinkle the cheese over the top of the frittata. Slide onto a plate, cut into 3 wedges, and serve. Leftovers can be covered, refrigerated overnight, and reheated in a microwave on reduced power.

NUTRITIONAL FACTS PER SERVING			
		Fat	7 g
		Sat Fat	2.5 g
Calories	120	Trans Fat	0 g
Protein	11 g	Cholesterol	130 mg
Carbohydrates	5 g	Phosphorus	146 mg
Fiber	1 g	Potassium	229 mg
		Sodium	200 mg

DIABETIC EXCHANGES

.19 starch
.33 meat (very lean)
.5 meat (lean)
.65 meat (medium fat)
.28 vegetable
.29 fat

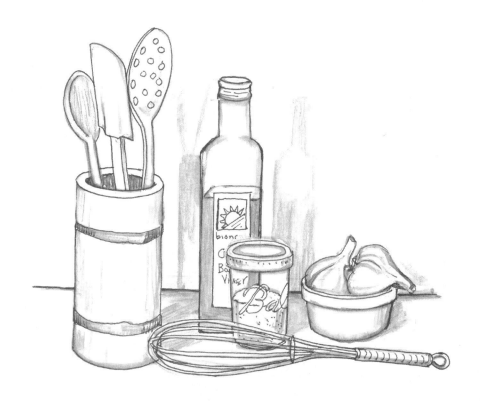

FOR:

- DASH Diet
- Diabetes Diet
- Dialysis Diet
- Heart Health Diet
- Kidney Stone Reduction Diet
- Low-Protein Diet
- Post-Transplant Diet
- Vegetarian Diet

BROCCOLI FRITTATA

Check with your doctor or dietitian to make sure that this recipe is compatible with your current dietary needs and limitations.

YIELD: 4 SERVINGS

• • • • • •

1 teaspoon olive or canola oil

1 cup chopped broccoli

$1/4$ cup thinly sliced onion

1 clove garlic, minced

4 large eggs

1 cup fat-free egg substitute

2 tablespoons water

$1/2$ cup shredded reduced-fat Cheddar cheese

1. Brush the oil over an oven-safe 12-inch nonstick skillet with sloping sides, and heat the skillet over medium heat. Preheat the broiler.

2. Place the broccoli, onion, and garlic in the skillet and sauté until the vegetables are tender. If the broccoli isn't cooking quickly enough, add a few tablespoons of water and cover to steam for a couple of minutes.

3. Place the eggs, egg substitute, and water in a large bowl, and whisk until well blended. Pour the egg mixture over the vegetable mixture in the skillet. Cook for 2 to 4 minutes or until the bottom is lightly browned. During cooking, lift the edges with a spatula and tilt the skillet from time to time so that the uncooked egg flows underneath.

4. Once the egg is set around the edges and starting to firm up in the middle, scatter the cheese over the top and transfer the skillet to the broiler. Cook for 3 to 5 minutes, or until the top is lightly browned and the mixture is firm to the touch. Rotate the skillet as necessary for even browning.

5. Remove the pan from the oven. Slide the frittata onto a plate, cut into 4 wedges, and serve. Leftovers can be covered, refrigerated overnight, and reheated in a microwave oven on reduced power.

NUTRITIONAL FACTS		Fat	9 g	DIABETIC EXCHANGES
PER SERVING		Sat Fat	3.5 g	• • • • • •
• • • • •		Trans Fat	0 g	.72 meat (lean)
Calories	160	Cholesterol	195 mg	.98 meat (medium fat)
Protein	17 g	Phosphorus	243 mg	.47 vegetable
Carbohydrates	4 g	Potassium	295 mg	.22 fats
Fiber	< 1 g	Sodium	300 mg	

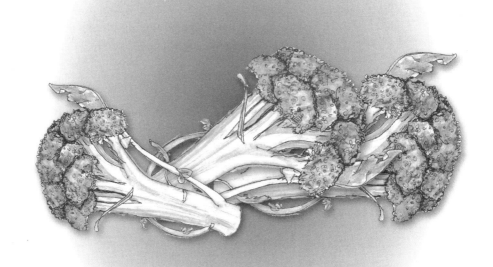

FOR:

- DASH Diet
- Diabetes Diet
- Dialysis Diet
- Heart Health Diet
- Kidney Stone
  Reduction Diet
- Low-Protein Diet
- Post-Transplant Diet
- Vegetarian Diet

BLUEBERRY BREAKFAST TREATS

Check with your doctor or dietitian to make sure that this recipe is compatible with your current dietary needs and limitations.

YIELD: 10 SERVINGS

• • • • • •

1 1/2 cups uncooked old-fashioned oats (cook in 5 minutes), divided

1 1/2 tablespoons sugar

1 teaspoon double-acting baking powder

1 1/2 tablespoons unsweetened applesauce

1/4 cup rice milk, plus additional to use as wash for treats

1/2 cup dried blueberries

2 tablespoons flour for cutting board

Glaze

1/4 cup confectioner's sugar

1 tablespoon rice milk

1/2 teaspoon vanilla extract

1/4 teaspoon ground cinnamon

1. Preheat the oven to 350°F. Line a large baking sheet (about 14 by 16 inches) with aluminum foil, spray the foil with cooking spray, and set aside.

2. To make the treats, place 1 cup of the oats plus the sugar and baking powder in a food processor, and pulse until the oats are the consistency of flour.

3. Add all of the applesauce and rice milk to the food processor, and pulse until the mixture is well blended and has the consistency of dough.

4. Sprinkle a little flour over a large cutting board. Turn the dough onto the floured surface, add the blueberries and all but 2 tablespoons of the remaining oats, and knead until the blueberries and oats are well mixed in.

5. Flatten the dough into an 8-inch wide disk, about 1/2 inch thick, and carefully transfer the dough to the prepared baking sheet. Brush a little rice milk over the top and sprinkle with the remaining 2 tablespoons of oats. Cut the dough into 10 wedges, leaving the wedges in place.

6. Bake the treats for 10 to 15 minutes, or until firm to the touch and lightly golden brown on the top. Remove the treats from the oven and allow to cool while you prepare the glaze.

7. Place all of the glaze ingredients in a small bowl, and mix with a whisk until smooth. Add more rice milk or sugar as necessary to get the right consistency. The glaze should be thick but should easily drizzle off the end of a fork.

8. Either use a fork to drizzle the glaze over the treats, or use a pastry brush to gently paint it over the tops. Allow to cool to room temperature, and serve.

NUTRITIONAL FACTS PER SERVING		Fat	1 g
		Sat Fat	0 g
• • • • •		Trans Fat	0 g
Calories	100	Cholesterol	0 mg
Protein	2 g	Phosphorus	63 mg
Carbohydrates	22 g	Potassium	63 mg
Fiber	2 g	Sodium	55 mg

DIABETIC EXCHANGES
• • • • • •
.62 starch
.43 fruit
.36 other carbs

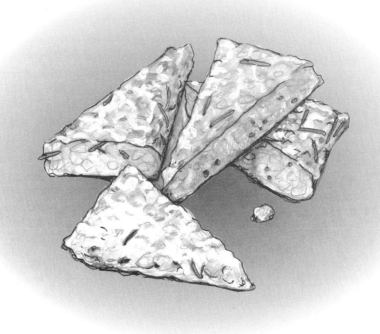

QUINOA SCRAMBLE

Check with your doctor or dietitian to make sure that this recipe is compatible with your current dietary needs and limitations.

YIELD: 2 SERVINGS

• • • • • •

I large egg

2 large egg whites

$^1/_2$ teaspoon freshly ground black pepper

$^1/_2$ tablespoon extra virgin olive oil

$^1/_2$ cup thinly sliced red bell pepper

I clove garlic, minced

I cup spinach

$^1/_2$ cup cooked quinoa

I tablespoon grated Parmesan cheese

1. Place the eggs and pepper in a small bowl, and whisk until well blended. Set aside.

2. Brush the oil over a 10-inch nonstick skillet, and heat over medium heat. Add the red pepper and garlic to the skillet, and cook until the red pepper is tender. Stir in the spinach, and cook for 1 minute, or until the spinach is wilted.

3. Add the egg mixture to the skillet, and cook, stirring constantly, until the eggs reach the desired consistency. Stir in the cooked quinoa, mixing well.

4. Transfer the scramble to a plate, top with the Parmesan cheese, and serve.

NUTRITIONAL FACTS PER SERVING			
• • • • •		Fat	8 g
		Sat Fat	2 g
		Trans Fat	0 g
Calories	160	Cholesterol	95 mg
Protein	10 g	Phosphorus	163 mg
Carbohydrates	13 g	Potassium	303 mg
Fiber	2 g	Sodium	150 mg

DIABETIC EXCHANGES
• • • • • •
.5 meat (very lean)
.67 meat (medium fat)
.5 vegetable
.66 fats

ENTRÉES

KUNG PAO CHICKEN

Check with your doctor or dietitian to make sure that this recipe is compatible with your current dietary needs and limitations.

YIELD: 6 SERVINGS

● ● ● ● ● ●

1 cup uncooked white rice

2 tablespoons red wine vinegar

2 teaspoons reduced-sodium soy sauce

2 teaspoons sugar

1 pound boneless, skinless chicken breast, cut into 1-inch pieces

1 tablespoon cornstarch

1 tablespoon olive oil

1 scallion, chopped, green tops only

2 cloves garlic, chopped

$3/_4$ teaspoon crushed red pepper flakes

$1/_2$ teaspoon grated fresh ginger

$1/_3$ cup dry-roasted peanuts, unsalted

1. Cook the rice according to package directions, omitting butter and salt.

2. While the rice is cooking, place the vinegar, soy sauce, and sugar in a small bowl. Stir together, and set aside.

3. Place the chicken in a medium-sized bowl. Sprinkle with the cornstarch, and toss to coat evenly.

4. Place the oil in a large skillet, and heat over medium-high heat. Add the chicken, and cook, stirring often, for 5 to 7 minutes, or until the chicken is no longer pink inside when cut with a knife. Transfer the chicken to a plate, and cover to keep warm.

5. Add the scallion, garlic, red pepper flakes, and ginger to the pan, and stir-fry for 15 seconds. Remove the pan from the heat and stir in the soy sauce mixture.

6. Stir the cooked chicken and the peanuts into the scallion mixture, and serve over the rice.

NUTRITIONAL FACTS PER SERVING			
		Fat	8 g
		Sat Fat	1.5 g
● ● ● ● ●		Trans Fat	0 g
Calories	280	Cholesterol	50 mg
Protein	20 g	Phosphorus	240 mg
Carbohydrates	31 g	Potassium	379 mg
Fiber	1 g	Sodium	150 mg

DIABETIC EXCHANGES
● ● ● ● ● ●
1.6 starch
2.7 meat (very lean)
1 fat

SHRIMP SCAMPI WITH PASTA

Check with your doctor or dietitian to make sure that this recipe is compatible with your current dietary needs and limitations.

YIELD: 3 SERVINGS

• • • • • •

3 ounces uncooked spaghetti

2 tablespoons olive oil, divided

$1/4$ cup finely chopped onion

$1/2$ cup frozen artichoke hearts, cooked and drained

$1/4$ cup dry white wine, such as Pinot Grigio

5 thin slices lemon, peeled

2 cloves garlic, minced

1 teaspoon crushed red pepper flakes

6 ounces cleaned, peeled large shrimp

1 teaspoon dried parsley

1. Cook the spaghetti according to package directions, omitting salt. Drain well, and cover to keep warm.

2. While the pasta is cooking, place 1 tablespoon of the olive oil in a large nonstick skillet, and heat over medium heat. Add the onion, mix, and cover. Reduce the heat to low-medium and cook until very soft. (Do not brown the onions.)

3. Add the artichoke hearts, white wine, lemon slices, garlic, and red pepper flakes to the pan, and cook uncovered for 5 to 7 minutes, or until the liquid is slightly reduced.

4. Add the shrimp, and cook, stirring occasionally, for 4 to 7 minutes, or until the shrimp are opaque inside when cut with a knife. Discard the lemon slices.

5. Stir the remaining tablespoon of olive oil and the parsley into the shrimp mixture. Divide the cooked spaghetti among 3 plates, and top with the shrimp mixture. Serve.

NUTRITIONAL FACTS PER SERVING			
• • • • •		Fat	11 g
		Sat Fat	1.5 g
		Trans Fat	0 g
Calories	290	Cholesterol	85 mg
Protein	17 g	Phosphorus	202 mg
Carbohydrates	29 g	Potassium	309 mg
Fiber	4 g	Sodium	105 mg

DIABETIC EXCHANGES
• • • • • •
1.3 starch
1.7 meat (very lean)
1 vegetable
2 fat

SPICY CHICKEN SANDWICH

Check with your doctor or dietitian to make sure that this recipe is compatible with your current dietary needs and limitations.

YIELD: I SERVING

• • • • • •

$^1/_2$ boneless, skinless chicken breast (3 ounces)

I plain dinner roll (about 1.5 ounces), split lengthwise

Marinade

2 tablespoons olive oil

I tablespoon red wine vinegar

$^1/_4$ teaspoon crushed red pepper flakes

$^1/_4$ teaspoon dried thyme, ground

1. Place all of the marinade ingredients in a small plastic bag with a zip-type closure, and shake to combine. Add the chicken, turn to coat, and place in the refrigerator to marinate overnight, occasionally turning the bag.

2. When you're ready to cook the chicken, preheat the oven to 350°F.

3. Spray a small nonstick skillet with cooking spray and heat over medium-high heat. Add the marinated chicken breast and cook for about 4 minutes on each side, or until the center of the chicken is no longer pink when cut with a knife.

4. Transfer the chicken to a plate, and shred the meat using 2 forks. Place the chicken on the split roll.

5. Place the sandwich on a small pan, and toast in the oven for 5 to 10 minutes, or until the bread is lightly browned. Serve.

NUTRITIONAL FACTS PER SERVING			
		Fat	32 g
		Sat Fat	4.5 g
• • • • •		Trans Fat	0 g
Calories	470	Cholesterol	55 mg
Protein	23 g	Phosphorus	234 mg
Carbohydrates	23 g	Potassium	392 mg
Fiber	I g	Sodium	330 mg

DIABETIC EXCHANGES
• • • • • •
1.6 starch
2.7 meat (very lean)
5.3 fat

CRUNCHY CHICKEN NUGGETS

Check with your doctor or dietitian to make sure that this recipe is compatible with your current dietary needs and limitations.

YIELD: 6 SERVINGS

• • • • • •

3 $^1/_2$ cups cornflakes

2 egg whites

2 tablespoons nonfat milk

$^1/_2$ teaspoon freshly ground black pepper

1 pound boneless, skinless chicken breast, cut into bite-size pieces

1. Preheat the oven to 400°F. Spray a large rimmed baking sheet with nonstick cooking spray, and set aside.

2. Place the cornflakes in a large plastic bag with a zip-type closure, and seal. Using a rolling pin or a can of food, crush the flakes until you have crumbs of a fairly uniform size. Do not crush to a fine powder. Set aside.

3. Place the egg whites, milk, and pepper in a small bowl, and whisk until well combined. Dip the chicken pieces in the egg mixture, coating them well with the egg. Then transfer the chicken to the bag of corn flake crumbs, seal the bag, and shake until the chicken is coated with the crumbs.

4. Arrange the chicken in a single layer on the prepared pan, and bake for 15 minutes, or until the chicken is no longer pink inside when cut with a sharp knife.

5. Serve the hot chicken nuggets immediately. If desired, add a dipping sauce such as Just Right Barbeque Sauce (see page 146).

NUTRITIONAL FACTS PER SERVING			
• • • • •		Fat	2 g
		Sat Fat	0 g
		Trans Fat	0 g
Calories	140	Cholesterol	45 mg
Protein	17 g	Phosphorus	210 mg
Carbohydrates	13 g	Potassium	256 mg
Fiber	0 g	Sodium	370 mg

DIABETIC EXCHANGES
• • • • • •
.71 starch
.2 meat (very lean)

SALMON WITH FRUIT SALSA

Check with your doctor or dietitian to make sure that this recipe is compatible with your current dietary needs and limitations.

YIELD: 6 SERVINGS

• • • • • • • •

6 (3-oz) salmon fillets, skin on

1 tablespoon plus 1 teaspoon olive oil

$^1/_2$ teaspoon freshly ground black pepper

Pineapple and Strawberry Salsa

$^1/_2$ cup diced pineapple

$^1/_4$ cup diced strawberries

$^1/_4$ cup diced red onion

1 jalapeño pepper, stemmed, seeded, and finely chopped

1 tablespoon chopped fresh mint

1 tablespoon chopped fresh cilantro

2 tablespoons fresh lemon juice

1 tablespoon fresh lime juice

1. To make the salsa, place all of the salsa ingredients in a small bowl, and stir to mix. Cover with plastic wrap and allow to sit at room temperature for 20 to 30 minutes so that the flavors blend.

2. Preheat a grill to medium.

3. Brush both sides of the salmon fillets with the olive oil, and season with the pepper. Place the fish on the grill, skin side down, and cook for about 3 minutes. Turn the fish 45 degrees and cook for an additional 3 minutes to create grill marks. Turn the fish over and cook for an additional 2 minutes, or until cooked through to the desired degree of doneness.

4. Arrange the fish on plates, topping each with some salsa. Serve immediately.

NUTRITIONAL FACTS PER SERVING			
		Fat	8 g
		Sat Fat	1.5 g
• • • • •		Trans Fat	0 g
Calories	160	Cholesterol	45 mg
Protein	17 g	Phosphorus	177 mg
Carbohydrates	4 g	Potassium	470 mg
Fiber	<1 g	Sodium	40 mg

DIABETIC EXCHANGES
• • • • • •
2.19 meat (lean)
.14 vegetable
.17 fruit
.59 fat

BEEF AND VEGETABLE STEW WITH RICE

Check with your doctor or dietitian to make sure that this recipe is compatible with your current dietary needs and limitations.

YIELD: 8 SERVINGS

• • • • • • • •

1 tablespoon vegetable oil

$3/_4$ cup chopped onion

3 garlic cloves, chopped

1 pound round steak, cut into $1/_2$-inch pieces

12 ounces canned no-salt-added diced tomatoes, undrained

1 tablespoon minced fresh parsley, or 1 teaspoon dried parsley

1 teaspoon dried basil leaves

$1/_2$ teaspoon dried thyme

$1/_4$ teaspoon freshly ground black pepper

2 cups thinly sliced green cabbage

1 cup sliced carrots

$3/_4$ cup frozen green peas

$1/_2$ cup sliced celery

$1/_2$ cup uncooked rice

1 cup water

1. Place the oil in a large heavy pot with a lid, and heat over medium-high heat. Add the onion and garlic, and sauté until soft.

2. Add the round steak to the pot and cook, stirring frequently, until the meat has browned.

3. Add the tomatoes, parsley, basil, thyme, and pepper. Cover and simmer for 45 to 60 minutes, or until the meat is tender, stirring occasionally.

4. Stir the cabbage, carrots, peas, celery, and rice into the meat mixture. Add the cup of water, and stir again.

5. Increase the heat to a boil. Then reduce the heat to a simmer, cover, and cook for 30 minutes, or until the vegetables and rice are tender. If the rice is too dry, add more water and cook until done. Serve.

NUTRITIONAL FACTS PER SERVING			
• • • • • •		Fat	8 g
		Sat Fat	3 g
		Trans Fat	0 g
Calories	210	Cholesterol	40 mg
Protein	14	Phosphorus	160 mg
Carbohydrates	19	Potassium	476 mg
Fiber	3 g	Sodium	55 mg

DIABETIC EXCHANGES
• • • • • •
.7 starch
2 meat (lean)
1.25 vegetable
.33 fat

FOR:
- DASH Diet
- Diabetes Diet
- Dialysis Diet
- Heart Health Diet
- Kidney Stone Reduction Diet
- Post-Transplant Diet

NOT FOR:
- Low-Protein Diet
- Vegetarian Diet

STEAK FAJITA PITA

Check with your doctor or dietitian to make sure that this recipe is compatible with your current dietary needs and limitations.

YIELD: 4 SERVINGS

• • • • • •

12 ounces flank steak, trimmed

1 tablespoon canola oil

1 small green bell pepper, chopped

2 tablespoons Italian Dressing (see page 148) or bottled low-salt Italian dressing

2 white pita rounds (about 6.5 inches in diameter), halved crosswise

1/4 cup lower-sodium salsa

1/4 cup shredded reduced-fat Cheddar cheese

1. Place the steak in the freezer for 15 minutes. Remove from the freezer and slice thinly across the grain.

2. Place the oil in a large nonstick pan, and heat over medium-high heat. Add the beef and green pepper, and sauté, stirring often, for about 2 minutes, or until the beef is no longer pink.

3. Transfer the steak and green pepper to a small bowl, and add the dressing. Toss to combine.

4. Fill each pita half with a quarter of the beef mixture, top with a tablespoon of salsa and a tablespoon of cheese, and serve.

NUTRITIONAL FACTS PER SERVING			
		Fat	17 g
		Sat Fat	4 g
• • • • •		Trans Fat	0 g
Calories	330	Cholesterol	55 mg
Protein	23 g	Phosphorus	251 mg
Carbohydrates	20 g	Potassium	406 mg
Fiber	1 g	Sodium	270 mg

DIABETIC EXCHANGES
• • • • • •
1 starch
3.5 meat (very lean)
.4 meat (lean)
.33 vegetable
2 fat

ROSEMARY CRUSTED PORK

Check with your doctor or dietitian to make sure that this recipe is compatible with your current dietary needs and limitations.

YIELD: 6 SERVINGS

• • • • • •

¹/₄ cup plain (unseasoned) breadcrumbs

2 cloves garlic, minced

1 tablespoon chopped fresh rosemary, or 1 teaspoon dried rosemary

¹/₂ teaspoon freshly ground black pepper

1 ¹/₄-pound pork tenderloin, trimmed

1 teaspoon olive oil

1. Preheat the oven to 425°F. Spray a large rimmed baking sheet with nonstick cooking spray, and set it aside.

2. Place the breadcrumbs, garlic, rosemary, and pepper in a small bowl, and stir to mix well. Set aside.

3. Rub the tenderloin with the olive oil. Then coat the tenderloin with the breadcrumb mixture.

4. Place the tenderloin on the prepared pan, and roast for 20 to 30 minutes, or until an instant-read thermometer registers an internal temperature of 145°F.

5. Remove the pan from the oven, and allow the roast to rest for 5 minutes. Slice thinly and serve.

NUTRITIONAL FACTS PER SERVING			
		Fat	3 g
		Sat Fat	1 g
• • • • •		Trans Fat	0 g
Calories	130	Cholesterol	60 mg
Protein	21 g	Phosphorus	243 mg
Carbohydrates	4 g	Potassium	394 mg
Fiber	0 g	Sodium	85 mg

DIABETIC EXCHANGES
• • • • • •
.25 starch
3.25 meat (very lean)
.15 fat

FOR:
- DASH Diet
- Diabetes Diet
- Dialysis Diet
- Heart Health Diet
- Kidney Stone
  Reduction Diet
- Post-Transplant Diet

NOT FOR:
- Low-Protein Diet
- Vegetarian Diet

PHILLY CHEESESTEAK

Check with your doctor or dietitian to make sure that this recipe is compatible with your current dietary needs and limitations.

YIELD: 4 SERVINGS

• • • • • •

12 ounces flank steak, trimmed

$1/_4$ teaspoon freshly ground black pepper

2 teaspoons olive oil, divided

$1^1/_2$ cups chopped green bell pepper

1 cup sliced onion

2 teaspoons chopped garlic

$1/_2$ teaspoon Worcestershire sauce

4 soft hoagie rolls with sesame seeds (about 2.3 ounces each)

4 slices reduced-fat "deli-style" Swiss cheese

1. Place the steak in the freezer for 15 minutes. Remove from the freezer and slice thinly across the grain. Sprinkle the slices with pepper, and set aside.

2. Preheat the oven broiler.

3. While the broiler is heating up, place 1 teaspoon of the oil in a large nonstick pan, and heat over medium-high heat. Add the beef and sauté, stirring often, for about 2 minutes, or until the beef is no longer pink. Remove the beef from the pan, and set aside.

4. Place the remaining oil in the pan and add the green pepper, onion, and garlic. Cook, stirring constantly, until the vegetables are tender.

5. Add the cooked beef and Worcestershire sauce to the pan, and stir to combine with the vegetables. Remove the pan from the heat.

6. Hollow out the top and bottom halves of the rolls, leaving a $1/_2$-inch-thick shell. Divide the steak mixture evenly among the roll bottoms, and top with the cheese. Place under the broiler just until the cheese is melted. Replace the tops of the hoagie rolls, and serve.

NUTRITIONAL FACTS PER SERVING				DIABETIC EXCHANGES
		Fat	18 g	
		Sat Fat	6 g	• • • • • •
• • • • •		Trans Fat	0 g	3.5 meat (very lean)
Calories	440	Cholesterol	65 mg	1 meat (lean)
Protein	33 g	Phosphorus	189 mg	1 vegetable
Carbohydrates	42 g	Potassium	424 mg	.5 fat
Fiber	3 g	Sodium	440 mg	

FOR:
- DASH Diet
- Diabetes Diet
- Dialysis Diet
- Heart Health Diet
- Kidney Stone
  Reduction Diet
- Low-Protein Diet
- Post-Transplant Diet
- Vegetarian Diet

MEXICAN LASAGNA

Check with your doctor or dietitian to make sure that this recipe is compatible with your current dietary needs and limitations.

YIELD: 12 SERVINGS

• • • • • •

4 small zucchini, sliced

1 small red bell pepper, cut into bite-size pieces

1 small green bell pepper, cut into bite-size pieces

1 large onion, chopped

28-ounce can no-salt-added whole tomatoes in tomato purée, undrained

8-ounce jar hot picante sauce

1 teaspoon ground cumin

1 pound uncooked lasagna noodles

15-ounce can reduced-sodium chickpeas, rinsed and drained

2 cups shredded low-fat Monterey Jack cheese

8 ounces fat-free sour cream

1. Steam the zucchini, bell peppers, and onion until tender. Spoon half of the vegetables into a bowl, and set aside. Transfer the remaining vegetables to a large skillet.

2. Stir the tomatoes, picante sauce, and cumin into the skillet mixture, and bring the mixture to a boil over high heat. Reduce the heat to low and simmer uncovered for 20 minutes, or until slightly thickened, stirring occasionally.

3. While the sauce is thickening, cook the lasagna noodles according to package directions, omitting salt. Drain well.

4. After the sauce has thickened, stir in the chickpeas. Preheat the oven to 375°F, and lightly oil a 14 x 10-inch casserole dish. Place $\frac{1}{2}$ cup of the shredded cheese in a small bowl, and set aside.

5. To assemble the lasagna, spoon $\frac{1}{2}$ cup of the sauce over the bottom of the prepared dish, spreading evenly. Evenly spread a third of the noodles over the sauce. Sprinkle a third of the cheese over the noodles. Spoon about a third of the sauce over the cheese. Repeat with the remaining ingredients, adding two more noodle-cheese-sauce layers. Spoon all of the sour cream evenly over the last sauce layer, and cover the dish loosely with aluminum foil.

6. Bake the lasagna for 35 minutes. Remove the foil and spoon the reserved vegetable mixture over the lasagna. Sprinkle with the reserved $\frac{1}{2}$ cup of cheese.

7. Bake uncovered for 10 minutes, or until heated through. Allow to sit for 5 minutes before cutting into 12 squares and serving.

NUTRITIONAL FACTS PER SERVING				
• • • • •				
Calories	290	Fat	5 g	
Protein	14 g	Sat Fat	2.5 g	
Carbohydrates	47 g	Trans Fat	0 g	
Fiber	4 g	Cholesterol	15 mg	
		Phosphorus	150 mg	
		Potassium	498 mg	
		Sodium	310 mg	

DIABETIC EXCHANGES

• • • • • •

2.2 starch
.8 meat (medium fat)
1.5 vegetable

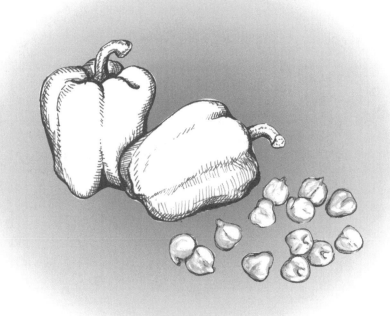

FOR:
- DASH Diet
- Diabetes Diet
- Dialysis Diet
- Heart Health Diet
- Kidney Stone Reduction Diet
- Low-Protein Diet
- Post-Transplant Diet

NOT FOR:
- Vegetarian Diet

SPICY PASTA

Check with your doctor or dietitian to make sure that this recipe is compatible with your current dietary needs and limitations.

YIELD: 2 SERVINGS

• • • • • •

4 ounces uncooked spaghetti

$1/2$ tablespoon olive oil

$1/3$ cup diced onion

$1/2$ cup no-salt-added canned tomato purée

$1/4$ cup reduced-sodium chicken or vegetable broth

I teaspoon garlic powder

I teaspoon crushed red pepper

1. Cook the spaghetti according to package directions, omitting salt. Drain well, and cover to keep warm.

2. While the pasta is cooking, place the olive oil in a large skillet, and heat over medium-high heat. Add the onion and cook, stirring occasionally, for about 5 minutes, or until the onion is tender.

3. Add the tomato purée, broth, garlic powder, and red pepper to the onions. Stir to combine, bring to a boil, and reduce the heat to a simmer.

4. Stir the cooked spaghetti into the tomato mixture, and serve immediately.

NUTRITIONAL FACTS PER SERVING			
• • • • •		Fat	4.5 g
		Sat Fat	.5 g
		Trans Fat	0 g
Calories	280	Cholesterol	0 mg
Protein	10 g	Phosphorus	157 mg
Carbohydrates	51 g	Potassium	500 mg
Fiber	4 g	Sodium	230 mg

DIABETIC EXCHANGES
• • • • • •
2.6 starch
1.35 vegetable
.7 fat

PESTO PASTA WITH VEGETABLES

Check with your doctor or dietitian to make sure that this recipe is compatible with your current dietary needs and limitations.

YIELD: 8 SERVINGS

• • • • • •

1 pound uncooked spaghetti

2 tablespoons olive oil

2 cups ¹/₂-inch cubes zucchini or yellow squash

1 pint cherry tomatoes

¹/₂ cup chopped onion

2 cloves garlic, chopped

7 ounces Basil Pesto (see page 147)

1. Cook the spaghetti according to package directions, omitting salt. Drain well, reserving ¹/₂ cup of the pasta cooking water.

2. While the pasta is cooking, heat the olive oil in a large skillet over medium heat. Add the zucchini, tomatoes, onion, and garlic, and sauté, stirring often, until the zucchini is crisp-tender and the cherry tomatoes begin to split. Set aside.

3. Return the drained pasta to the pot. Add the pesto, and toss to mix. Add the vegetable mixture, and cook a minute or two over high heat, adding a tablespoon or two of pasta water to loosen the sauce, if necessary. Serve immediately.

NUTRITIONAL FACTS PER SERVING			
		Fat	14 g
		Sat Fat	2 g
• • • • • •		Trans Fat	0 g
Calories	350	Cholesterol	<5 mg
Protein	11 g	Phosphorus	197 mg
Carbohydrates	47 g	Potassium	370 mg
Fiber	3 g	Sodium	70 mg

DIABETIC EXCHANGES
• • • • • •
2.6 starch
.2 meat (medium fat)
.8 vegetable
2.25 fat

TOFU CHILI

Check with your doctor or dietitian to make sure that this recipe is compatible with your current dietary needs and limitations.

YIELD: 3 SERVINGS

• • • • • •

6 ounces frozen firm tofu, thawed

2 tablespoons water

2 tablespoons vegetable oil, divided

1 tablespoon lower-sodium soy sauce

$1\frac{1}{2}$ teaspoons no-salt-added tomato paste

$\frac{1}{4}$ teaspoon onion powder

$\frac{1}{4}$ teaspoon garlic powder

1 small green pepper, diced

1 small onion, diced

1 clove garlic, minced

1 medium tomato, diced

$\frac{1}{2}$ cup cooked chickpeas, with liquid, or canned low-sodium chickpeas

$2\frac{1}{2}$ teaspoons chili powder

$\frac{1}{4}$ teaspoon ground cumin

1. Place the thawed tofu between paper towels, or wrap it in a clean kitchen towel. Using your hands, press out as much excess water at possible. Tear the tofu into bite-sized pieces, and set aside.

2. Place the water, $1\frac{1}{2}$ teaspoons of the vegetable oil, and all of the soy sauce, tomato paste, onion powder, and garlic powder in a medium-size bowl, and mix to combine. Add the tofu to the soy sauce mixture, and mix well until all pieces are evenly coated.

3. Place a tablespoon of the oil in a deep skillet, and heat over medium heat. Add the tofu mixture, and cook, stirring often, until the tofu is well browned. Leave the tofu in the pan, and set aside.

4. Place the remaining $1\frac{1}{2}$ teaspoons of oil in a separate skillet, and heat over medium-high heat. Add the green pepper, onion, and garlic, and cook, stirring often, until the onion is transparent and the green pepper has softened.

5. Add the sautéed vegetables, tomato, chickpeas, chili powder, and cumin to the tofu, and stir to mix. Add water as needed to cover.

6. Bring the mixture to a simmer, and simmer for 5 minutes. Serve immediately.

NUTRITIONAL FACTS		Fat	15
PER SERVING		Sat Fat	1.5 g
• • • • •		Trans Fat	0 g
Calories	240	Cholesterol	0 mg
Protein	13	Phosphorus	174 mg
Carbohydrates	18 g	Potassium	493 mg
Fiber	5	Sodium	220 mg

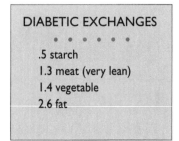

DIABETIC EXCHANGES
• • • • • •
.5 starch
1.3 meat (very lean)
1.4 vegetable
2.6 fat

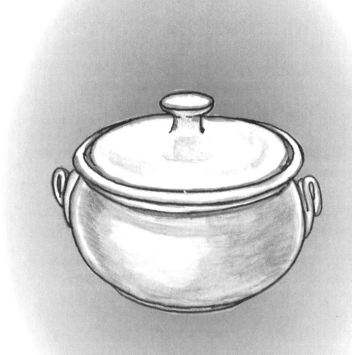

FOR:
■ DASH Diet
■ Diabetes Diet
■ Dialysis Diet
■ Heart Health Diet
■ Low-Protein Diet
■ Post-Transplant Diet
■ Vegetarian Diet
NOT FOR:
■ Kidney Stone
Reduction Diet

CURRIED TOFU WITH PEAS

Check with your doctor or dietitian to make sure that this recipe is compatible with your current dietary needs and limitations.

YIELD: 6 SERVINGS

• • • • • •

1 tablespoon olive oil

1 medium onion, diced

3 cloves garlic, minced

1 teaspoon minced fresh ginger

1 small jalapeño pepper, chopped

14 ounces frozen firm tofu, thawed, rinsed, and crumbled

1 teaspoon curry powder

1 cup frozen peas

2 teaspoons chopped cilantro (optional)

1. Place the olive oil in a large nonstick skillet with a cover, and heat over medium heat. Add the onion to the pan, and cook, stirring occasionally, for 5 to 7 minutes, or until the onion turns light golden brown. Add the garlic, ginger, and jalapeño pepper, and cook for 3 additional minutes.

2. Add the crumbled tofu and curry powder to the skillet, and stir well to combine. Reduce the heat to medium-low, and cover the pan. Cook for about 15 minutes, stirring often so that the tofu does not stick to the bottom of the skillet.

3. Stir the peas into the tofu mixture, and cook uncovered for 5 to 10 minutes. Remove from the heat, and, if desired, stir in the cilantro. Serve immediately with white rice or bread

NUTRITIONAL FACTS PER SERVING			
• • • • •			
Calories	90	Fat	8 g
Protein	11 g	Sat Fat	1 g
Carbohydrates	6 g	Trans Fat	0 g
Fiber	1 g	Cholesterol	0 mg
		Phosphorus	111 mg
		Potassium	201 mg
		Sodium	15 mg

DIABETIC EXCHANGES
• • • • • •
1 meat (lean)
.5 vegetable
.5 fat

PEPPER, ONION, AND ZUCCHINI PIZZA

Check with your doctor or dietitian to make sure that this recipe is compatible with your current dietary needs and limitations.

YIELD: 4 SERVINGS (2 SLICES EACH)

• • • • • •

2 tablespoons olive oil

1 bell pepper, any color, cut into $1/4$-inch strips

1 white or yellow onion, cut into $1/4$-inch strips

1 medium (5–6 inch) zucchini or yellow squash, cut into $1/4$-inch rounds

1 clove garlic, minced

1 frozen par-baked pizza crust, such as Trader Joe's Organic Pizza Crust

$1/2$ cup Spaghetti Sauce (see page 144)

1. Preheat the oven to 450°F. Line a large baking sheet with aluminum foil, and spray with nonstick cooking spray. Set aside.

2. Heat the olive oil in a large skillet over medium heat. Add the bell pepper, onion, zucchini, and garlic, and cook, stirring often, until the vegetables have softened and some are golden brown. Set aside.

3. While the vegetables are cooking, place the pizza crust on the prepared pan. Top with the Spaghetti Sauce, spreading it evenly but leaving a $1/2$-inch border around the crust. Arrange the sautéed vegetables over the sauce.

4. Bake for 10 to 15 minutes, or until the rim of the crust is lightly browned. Avoid burning.

5. Remove the pizza from the oven, and allow it to sit for 5 minutes. Cut into 8 slices, and serve immediately.

NUTRITIONAL FACTS PER SERVING				DIABETIC EXCHANGES
		Fat	16 g	• • • • • •
		Sat Fat	1 g	
• • • • •		Trans Fat	0 g	2 starch
Calories	320	Cholesterol	0 mg	1.5 vegetable
Protein	6 g	Phosphorus	60 mg*	2.5 fat
Carbohydrates	40 g	Potassium	396 mg*	
Fiber	4 g	Sodium	75 mg	

*The phosphorus and potassium data presented for this recipe were calculated using one brand of par-baked pizza crust. Because these nutrients can vary from brand to brand, contact the manufacturer of the pizza crust you choose to determine if that brand will meet your nutritional needs.

CURRIED CHICKEN BREAST

Check with your doctor or dietitian to make sure that this recipe is compatible with your current dietary needs and limitations.

YIELD: 8 SERVINGS

• • • • • •

1 tablepoon olive oil

1 large onion, chopped

4 cloves garlic, chopped

1 teaspoon grated fresh ginger

1 large tomato, chopped

8-ounce can no-salt-added tomato sauce

1 jalapeño pepper, chopped (optional)

1 teaspoon curry powder

1 teaspoon ground turmeric

1½ pounds boneless, skinless chicken breast, cut into 1-inch pieces

Chopped fresh cilantro (optional, for garnish)

1. Place the oil in a large skillet with a lid, and heat over medium-high heat. Add the onion and cook, stirring occasionally, until golden brown.

2. Add the garlic and ginger to the pan, and cook for 2 minutes.

3. Add the tomato, tomato sauce, jalapeño pepper, curry powder, and turmeric to the pan, and stir to mix well. Stir in the chicken.

4. Cover and cook over medium heat, stirring frequently to avoid burning, for about 15 minutes, or until the chicken is no longer pink inside when cut with a knife. Serve, sprinkling each serving with chopped cilantro, if desired.

NUTRITIONAL FACTS PER SERVING			
		Fat	3.5 g
		Sat Fat	.5 g
• • • • •		Trans Fat	0 g
Calories	130	Cholesterol	50 mg
Protein	20 g	Phosphorus	211 mg
Carbohydrates	5 g	Potassium	395 mg
Fiber	1 g	Sodium	50 mg

DIABETIC EXCHANGES
• • • • • • •
2.67 meat (very lean)
1 vegetable
.33 fat

SIDE DISHES
AND SALADS

FOR:
- DASH Diet
- Diabetes Diet
- Dialysis Diet
- Heart Health Diet
- Kidney Stone
  Reduction Diet
- Low-Protein Diet
- Post-Transplant Diet
- Vegetarian Diet

SHALLOT, GARLIC, AND LEMON GREEN BEANS

Check with your doctor or dietitian to make sure that this recipe is compatible with your current dietary needs and limitations.

YIELD: 6 SERVINGS

. . . . . .

1 pound green beans, trimmed

2 tablespoons olive oil

2 cloves garlic, minced

2 large shallots, thinly sliced

$1/2$ teaspoon freshly ground pepper

1 tablespoon fresh lemon juice

1. Bring a large pot of water to a boil over high heat. Drop in the green beans, and blanch until the beans are bright green in color and tender-crisp, approximately 2 minutes. Drain the beans and place them in a large bowl of ice water to stop the cooking. Leave in the ice water for about 2 minutes, or until the beans are cool to the touch. Drain the beans and set aside.

2. Place the olive oil in a large skillet and heat over medium-low heat. Add the garlic and shallots, and cook until soft and translucent.

3. Add the drained green beans and ground pepper to the pan, and cook, stirring frequently, for about 2 minutes, or until the beans are heated through.

4. Remove the pan from the heat, stir in the lemon juice, and serve immediately.

NUTRITIONAL FACTS PER SERVING			
. . . . . .		Fat	4.5 g
		Sat Fat	.5 g
		Trans Fat	0 g
Calories	70	Cholesterol	0 mg
Protein	2 g	Phosphorus	31 mg
Carbohydrates	6 g	Potassium	173 mg
Fiber	2 g	Sodium	5 mg

DIABETIC EXCHANGES
. . . . . .
.84 vegetable
.88 fat

FOR:

- DASH Diet
- Diabetes Diet
- Dialysis Diet
- Heart Health Diet
- Kidney Stone
  Reduction Diet
- Low-Protein Diet
- Post-Transplant Diet
- Vegetarian Diet

RICE WITH CORN AND SCALLIONS

Check with your doctor or dietitian to make sure that this recipe is compatible with your current dietary needs and limitations.

YIELD: 6 SERVINGS

• • • • • •

1 cup uncooked white rice

1 cup frozen yellow corn kernels, microwaved without salt or butter, or 1 cup fresh corn kernels

1 medium-size scallion, chopped

Dressing

2 tablespoons fresh lemon juice

2 tablespoons olive oil

1 tablespoon grated lemon zest

$\frac{1}{2}$ teaspoon freshly ground black pepper

1. Cook the rice according to package directions, omitting butter and salt.

2. While the rice is cooking, prepare the dressing by placing the dressing ingredients in a small bowl and whisking to combine. Set aside.

3. Place the prepared rice, corn, and scallion in a medium-size bowl, and toss to combine. Add the prepared dressing, and toss to coat evenly. Serve hot, at room temperature, or cold.

NUTRITIONAL FACTS PER SERVING			
		Fat	4.5 g
		Sat Fat	.5 g
• • • • •		Trans Fat	0 g
Calories	180	Cholesterol	0 mg
Protein	3 g	Phosphorus	53 mg
Carbohydrates	31 g	Potassium	92 mg
Fiber	1 g	Sodium	0 mg

DIABETIC EXCHANGES
• • • • • •
1.71 starch
.88 fat

FOR:
■ DASH Diet
■ Diabetes Diet
■ Dialysis Diet
■ Heart Health Diet
■ Kidney Stone
   Reduction Diet
■ Low-Protein Diet
■ Post-Transplant Diet
■ Vegetarian Diet

CREOLE CORN

Check with your doctor or dietitian to make sure that this recipe is compatible with your current dietary needs and limitations.

YIELD: 6 SERVINGS

• • • • • • • •

1 tablespoon olive oil

$1/4$ cup chopped onion

$1/4$ cup chopped green bell pepper

$1/4$ cup chopped red bell pepper

10 ounces fresh, frozen, or canned no-salt-added corn kernels, drained

$1/4$ cup diced fresh tomatoes or canned no-salt-added tomatoes, drained

1 tablespoon chopped fresh parsley

$1/4$ teaspoon freshly ground black pepper

$1/4$ teaspoon ground cumin

1. Place the olive oil in a 12-inch skillet, and heat over medium-high heat. Add the onion and peppers, and sauté, stirring occasionally, until the vegetables are tender.

2. Lower the heat to medium, and add all of the remaining ingredients, stirring to combine. Continue to cook until heated through, and serve immediately.

NUTRITIONAL FACTS PER SERVING			
• • • • •		Fat	2.5 g
		Sat Fat	0 g
		Trans Fat	0 g
Calories	70	Cholesterol	0 mg
Protein	2 g	Phosphorus	48 mg
Carbohydrates	13 g	Potassium	197 mg
Fiber	2 g	Sodium	0 mg

DIABETIC EXCHANGES
• • • • • •
.58 starch
.3 vegetable
.44 fat

CHOPPED SALAD

Check with your doctor or dietitian to make sure that this recipe is compatible with your current dietary needs and limitations.

YIELD: 8 SERVINGS

• • • • • • • •

3 cups chopped romaine lettuce

1 tomato, seeded and diced

$^1/_2$ cup canned no-salt-added red beans, rinsed and drained

$^1/_2$ cup canned no-salt-added chickpeas, rinsed and drained

$^1/_4$ cup shredded reduced-sodium Cheddar cheese

$^1/_4$ cup shredded reduced-sodium Monterey Jack cheese

Dressing

1 $^1/_2$ tablespoons balsamic vinegar

$^1/_2$ teaspoon Dijon mustard

$^1/_4$ teaspoon freshly ground black pepper

3 tablespoons olive oil

1. To make the dressing, place the vinegar, mustard, and pepper in a small bowl, and whisk until well mixed. Add the olive oil, and whisk until the dressing is emulsified. Set aside.

2. Place the romaine and remaining salad ingredients in a large bowl, and toss to mix. Add the salad dressing, and toss to coat. Serve immediately.

NUTRITIONAL FACTS PER SERVING			
		Fat	7 g
		Sat Fat	1.5 g
• • • • •		Trans Fat	0 g
Calories	110	Cholesterol	<5 mg
Protein	4 g	Phosphorus	79 mg
Carbohydrates	7 g	Potassium	165 mg
Fiber	2 g	Sodium	55 mg

DIABETIC EXCHANGES
• • • • • •
.34 starch
.1 meat (very lean)
.15 meat (medium fat)
.25 vegetable
1 fat

FOR:
- DASH Diet
- Diabetes Diet
- Dialysis Diet
- Heart Health Diet
- Kidney Stone Reduction Diet
- Low-Protein Diet
- Post-Transplant Diet
- Vegetarian Diet

FRUIT, NUT, AND GRAIN SALAD

Check with your doctor or dietitian to make sure that this recipe is compatible with your current dietary needs and limitations.

YIELD: 2 SERVINGS

• • • • • •

3 cups hand-shredded green leaf lettuce

$1/4$ cup cooked couscous

2 tablespoons sweetened dried cranberries, such as Craisins

$1/8$ cup dry-roasted almonds (unsalted)

Dressing

2 tablespoons olive oil

2 tablespoons balsamic vinegar

$1 1/2$ teaspoons honey

Pinch freshly ground black pepper

1. To make the dressing, place the dressing ingredients in a small bowl and whisk until well blended. Set aside.

2. Place the lettuce and couscous in a medium-size bowl, and toss to mix. Add the salad dressing, and toss to coat.

3. Divide the salad between two serving plates, and top each serving with half of the cranberries and nuts. Serve immediately.

NUTRITIONAL FACTS PER SERVING			
• • • • •		Fat	18 g
		Sat Fat	2 g
		Trans Fat	0 g
Calories	260	Cholesterol	0 mg
Protein	3 g	Phosphorus	64 mg
Carbohydrates	21 g	Potassium	200 mg
Fiber	2 g	Sodium	20 mg

DIABETIC EXCHANGES
• • • • • •
.3 starch
.27 meat (very lean)
.32 vegetable
.41 fruit
3.58 fat
.3 other carbs

136

TABBOULEH

Check with your doctor or dietitian to make sure that this recipe is compatible with your current dietary needs and limitations.

YIELD: 4 SERVINGS

• • • • • •

$1/_2$ cup uncooked bulgur wheat

3 tablespoons olive oil

1 cup water

1 plum tomato, cored and chopped into bite-size pieces

$1/_2$ cup chopped fresh parsley

$1/_3$ cucumber (unpeeled), chopped into bite-size pieces

3 tablespoons fresh lemon juice

$1/_4$ teaspoon freshly ground black pepper

1. Place the bulgur wheat in a large heatproof bowl. Add the olive oil, and stir to combine. Set aside.

2. Bring the water to a boil and carefully pour over the wheat mixture. Stir to mix, cover with plastic wrap, and allow to stand for 15 minutes, or until the wheat is soft.

3. Add the tomato, parsley, and cucumber to the wheat mixture, and stir to combine. Add the lemon juice and pepper, and toss to mix well. Cover and chill for at least an hour before serving.

NUTRITIONAL FACTS PER SERVING		Fat	11g
		Sat Fat	1.5 g
• • • • •		Trans Fat	0 g
Calories	160	Cholesterol	0 mg
Protein	3 g	Phosphorus	68 mg
Carbohydrates	16 g	Potassium	200 mg
Fiber	4 g	Sodium	10 mg

DIABETIC EXCHANGES
• • • • • • •
.75 starch
.37 vegetable
2 fat

137

FOR:
- DASH Diet
- Diabetes Diet
- Dialysis Diet
- Heart Health Diet
- Kidney Stone Reduction Diet
- Low-Protein Diet
- Post-Transplant Diet
- Vegetarian Diet

VEGETABLE AND BARLEY SALAD

Check with your doctor or dietitian to make sure that this recipe is compatible with your current dietary needs and limitations.

YIELD: 3 SERVINGS

· · · · · · · ·

1 1/4 cups water

1/2 cup uncooked pearl barley

1/4 cup chopped (unpeeled) cucumber

1/2 small red bell pepper, chopped

1 medium stalk celery, chopped

1 ounce feta cheese, crumbled (about 1/4 cup)

Dressing

3 tablespoons fresh lemon juice

1 teaspoon olive oil

2 leaves fresh basil, chopped

1/4 teaspoon garlic powder

1/4 teaspoon dried thyme

1. Place the water in a medium-sized saucepan and bring to a boil. Stir in the barley, reduce the heat to a simmer, and cover. Cook for about 30 minutes, or until the barley has absorbed all the water and is tender but still chewy. Remove from the heat and allow to cool for about 10 minutes.

2. While the barley is cooling, place the dressing ingredients in a small bowl and whisk until well mixed. Set aside.

3. Place the cucumber, red pepper, and celery in a large bowl. Add the prepared dressing, and toss to mix. Toss in the slightly cooled barley and the feta. Serve immediately, or cover and store in the refrigerator until ready to serve.

NUTRITIONAL FACTS PER SERVING			
		Fat	4 g
		Sat Fat	1.5 g
· · · · ·		Trans Fat	0 g
Calories	170	Cholesterol	10 mg
Protein	5 g	Phosphorus	117 mg
Carbohydrates	29 g	Potassium	194 mg
Fiber	6 g	Sodium	120 mg

DIABETIC EXCHANGES
· · · · · ·
1.5 starch
.25 meat (high fat)
.26 vegetable
.3 fat

FOR:
- DASH Diet
- Diabetes Diet
- Heart Health Diet
- Kidney Stone Reduction Diet
- Low-Protein Diet
- Post-Transplant Diet
- Vegetarian Diet

NOT FOR:
- Dialysis Diet

QUINOA WITH BRUSSELS SPROUTS

Check with your doctor or dietitian to make sure that this recipe is compatible with your current dietary needs and limitations.

YIELD: 6 SERVINGS

• • • • • • • •

2 cups low-sodium vegetable broth

$3/4$ cup uncooked quinoa

I teaspoon ground cumin

I teaspoon ground turmeric

I tablespoon plus I teaspoon ground coriander, divided

$1/4$ teaspoon freshly ground black pepper, divided

2 tablespoons olive oil

2 cloves garlic, minced

$1/2$ teaspoon smoked paprika

8 ounces Brussels sprouts, trimmed and shredded or thinly sliced

1. Place the broth, quinoa, cumin, turmeric, 1 teaspoon of the coriander, and $1/8$ teaspoon of the pepper in a saucepan, and bring the mixture to a boil. Turn the heat down to a simmer and cook until the quinoa starts to float in the water, 5 to 10 minutes. Turn the heat off, cover, and allow the quinoa to steam for 10 minutes. Stir the mixture once, and set it aside.

2. Place the oil and garlic in a large skillet, and cook over medium heat for about 20 seconds, or until the garlic is golden brown.

3. Add the smoked paprika, the remaining tablespoon of coriander, and the remaining $1/8$ teaspoon of pepper to the skillet, and cook for another 10 seconds. Stir in the Brussels sprouts, and cook for about 1 minute. Stir in the reserved cooked quinoa, and cook for another 30 seconds. Serve immediately.

NUTRITIONAL FACTS PER SERVING		Fat	7 g
		Sat Fat	I g
• • • • •		Trans Fat	0 g
Calories	150	Cholesterol	0 mg
Protein	6 g	Phosphorus	152 mg
Carbohydrates	19 g	Potassium	380 mg
Fiber	3 g	Sodium	35 mg

DIABETIC EXCHANGES
• • • • • •
I starch
.7 vegetable
.88 fat

BARBEQUE CHICKEN AND RICE SALAD

Check with your doctor or dietitian to make sure that this recipe is compatible with your current dietary needs and limitations.

YIELD: 3 SERVINGS

• • • • • • •

$1/_2$ boneless, skinless chicken breast (3 to 4 ounces)

1 cup cooked white rice (cooked without butter or salt), cooled

$1/_3$ cup canned no-salt-added black beans, rinsed and drained

2 tablespoons Just Right Barbeque Sauce (see page 146) or commercial low-sodium barbecue sauce

$1/_2$ cup fresh or canned no-salt-added yellow corn kernels, drained

1 scallion, chopped (greens only)

1. Place the chicken in a shallow pan, cover with water, and bring to a simmer. Cover and simmer for about 20 minutes or until the internal temperature of the chicken reaches 165°F. Remove the chicken from the water and allow to cool slightly.

2. Using two forks, shred the chicken. Set aside.

3. Place the rice and beans in a medium-size bowl, and add the barbeque sauce. Toss to coat.

4. Add the shredded chicken, corn, and scallion to the rice mixture, and toss to combine. Serve.

NUTRITIONAL FACTS PER SERVING			
		Fat	1.5 g
		Sat Fat	0 g
• • • • •		Trans Fat	0 g
Calories	180	Cholesterol	25 mg
Protein	12 g	Phosphorus	158 mg
Carbohydrates	29 g	Potassium	332 mg
Fiber	3 g	Sodium	55 mg

DIABETIC EXCHANGES
• • • • • •
1.6 starch
1.24 meat (very lean)
.13 vegetable

FOR:

- DASH Diet
- Diabetes Diet
- Dialysis Diet
- Heart Health Diet
- Kidney Stone Reduction Diet
- Low-Protein Diet
- Post-Transplant Diet
- Vegetarian Diet

ROASTED CAULIFLOWER

Check with your doctor or dietitian to make sure that this recipe is compatible with your current dietary needs and limitations.

YIELD: 4 SERVINGS

• • • • • •

1 small head cauliflower (about 9 ounces), cut into bite-size florets

3 tablespoons olive oil

1 tablespoon fresh lemon juice

2 cloves garlic, minced

$1/4$ teaspoon freshly ground black pepper

1. Preheat the oven to 425°F. Line a large baking sheet with parchment, or spray the sheet with nonstick cooking spray. Set aside.

2. Place the cauliflower, olive oil, lemon juice, garlic, and pepper in a large bowl, and toss until the cauliflower is lightly coated.

3. Arrange the cauliflower mixture in a single layer on the prepared baking sheet, and roast in the preheated oven for 16 to 20 minutes, or until the cauliflower is tender and lightly browned. Serve immediately.

NUTRITIONAL FACTS PER SERVING			
• • • • •			
Calories	110	Fat	10 g
Protein	1 g	Sat Fat	1.5 g
Carbohydrates	4 g	Trans Fat	0 g
Fiber	1 g	Cholesterol	0 mg
		Phosphorus	32 mg
		Potassium	200 mg
		Sodium	20 mg

DIABETIC EXCHANGES
• • • • • •
.75 vegetable
2 fats

SAUCES
AND SALAD
DRESSINGS

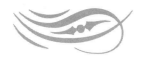

SPAGHETTI SAUCE

This sauce has a relatively high potassium count due to the tomatoes. Check with your doctor or dietitian to make sure that this recipe is compatible with your current dietary needs and limitations.

YIELD: 4 SERVINGS

• • • • • •

1 tablespoon olive oil

$^1/_2$ large onion, chopped

1 clove garlic, minced

15-ounce can no-salt-added crushed tomatoes

3 tablespoons no-salt-added tomato paste

$^1/_2$ teaspoon dried basil

$^1/_2$ teaspoon dried marjoram

$^1/_2$ teaspoon dried thyme

$^1/_2$ teaspoon freshly ground black pepper

1. Place the olive oil in a large skillet, and heat over medium-low heat. Add the onion and cook, stirring often, until the onion is transparent. Add the garlic and cook for an additional minute, or until fragrant.

2. Add the crushed tomatoes, tomato paste, basil, marjoram, and thyme to the pan, and stir to combine. Add the pepper to taste.

3. Adjust the heat to a simmer, and cook uncovered for 30 minutes, stirring occasionally. Serve the sauce over pasta, pizza, chicken, or pork.

NUTRITIONAL FACTS PER SERVING					DIABETIC EXCHANGES
		Fat	3.5 g		• • • • • •
		Sat Fat	0 g		2 vegetable
• • • • •		Trans Fat	0 g		.66 fat
Calories	80	Cholesterol	0 mg		
Protein	3 g	Phosphorus	123 mg		
Carbohydrates	10 g	Potassium	460 mg		
Fiber	3 g	Sodium	10 mg		

CHICKEN PASTA SAUCE

This sauce has a relatively high potassium count due to the tomatoes and chicken. Check with your doctor or dietitian to make sure that this recipe is compatible with your current dietary needs and limitations.

YIELD: 8 SERVINGS

• • • • • •

2 teaspoons olive oil

$1/2$ cup chopped onion

1 large carrot, chopped

1 large celery stalk, chopped

1 pound ground chicken

$1/4$ teaspoon freshly ground black pepper

28-ounce can no-salt-added crushed tomatoes

1 bay leaf

1. Place the olive oil in a large skillet, and heat over medium-high heat. Add the onion, carrot, and celery, and cook, stirring often, for about 5 minutes, or until the vegetables are soft.

2. Add the ground chicken and pepper to the skillet, and cook, stirring often to crumble, until the meat has browned.

3. Add the crushed tomatoes to the skillet, and continue to cook uncovered for 10 to 15 minutes, or until the sauce has thickened slightly.

4. Add the bay leaf, cover, and reduce the heat to a simmer. Cook, stirring the sauce occasionally, for about 1 hour. Remove and discard the bay leaf, and serve the sauce over pasta.

NUTRITIONAL FACTS PER SERVING			
• • • • •			
Calories	130	Fat	6 g
Protein	12 g	Sat Fat	1.5 g
Carbohydrates	7 g	Trans Fat	0 g
Fiber	2 g	Cholesterol	50 mg
		Phosphorus	207 mg
		Potassium	637 mg
		Sodium	45 mg

DIABETIC EXCHANGES
• • • • • •
1.67 vegetable
.22 fat

FOR:

■ DASH Diet
■ Diabetes Diet
■ Dialysis Diet
■ Heart Health Diet
■ Kidney Stone
  Reduction Diet
■ Low-Protein Diet
■ Post-Transplant Diet
■ Vegetarian Diet

JUST RIGHT BARBEQUE SAUCE

Check with your doctor or dietitian to make sure that this recipe is compatible with your current dietary needs and limitations.

YIELD: 22 SERVINGS (ABOUT 2 TABLESPOONS EACH)

• • • • • • • •

$1/2$ cup no-salt-added tomato paste

$1/4$ cup distilled white vinegar

$1 1/2$ cups water

$1/2$ cup finely chopped onion

2 tablespoons reduced-sodium Worcestershire sauce

2 tablespoons fresh lemon juice

2 tablespoons brown sugar

1 tablespoon paprika

1 tablespoon dried parsley

1 teaspoon dry mustard

$1/4$ teaspoon chili powder

$1/8$ teaspoon cayenne pepper

1 tablespoon cornstarch stirred into 2 tablespoons water until smooth

1. Place the tomato paste and vinegar in a large saucepan, and stir until well blended. Slowly stir in the water.

2. Add all of the remaining ingredients except for the cornstarch mixture, stirring thoroughly until blended.

3. Bring the mixture to a boil, and whisk in the cornstarch mixture. Reduce the heat to a simmer and cook for about 5 minutes, or until slightly thickened, stirring occasionally. Use to baste meat while grilling or to add flavor to sandwiches. Store any leftover sauce in a covered container in the refrigerator for up to 2 weeks.

NUTRITIONAL FACTS PER SERVING		Fat	0 g
		Sat Fat	0 g
• • • • •		Trans Fat	0 g
Calories	15	Cholesterol	0 mg
Protein	0 g	Phosphorus	8 mg
Carbohydrates	3 g	Potassium	90 mg
Fiber	0 g	Sodium	20 mg

DIABETIC EXCHANGES
• • • • • •
.27 vegetable

BASIL PESTO

Check with your doctor or dietitian to make sure that this recipe is compatible with your current dietary needs and limitations.

YIELD: 6 SERVINGS (ABOUT 1/4 CUP EACH)

• • • • • •

1/2 cup shelled pine nuts (pignoli)

4 cups fresh basil leaves

1/2 cup grated Parmesan cheese

1 1/2 tablespoons chopped garlic

1/4 cup extra virgin olive oil

2 tablespoons water

1. Heat a skillet over medium heat. Add the pine nuts, and cook, stirring constantly, until they are fragrant and golden brown on all sides. Be careful to avoid burning. Transfer the nuts to a plate to cool.

2. Place the basil, cooled pine nuts, Parmesan cheese, and garlic in a food processor. (Leave out the cheese if you plan to freeze the pesto.) Pulse, slowly adding the olive oil and water until you have the desired consistency. Scrape down the sides of the food processor as needed.

3. Use to dress pasta or to top vegetables, fish, chicken, or pizza. Store any leftover pesto in a covered container in the refrigerator for up to a week, or in the freezer for 3 to 4 months. If storing in the freezer, thaw the pesto and stir in the cheese before using.

NUTRITIONAL FACTS PER SERVING			
		Fat	19 g
		Sat Fat	3 g
• • • • • •		Trans Fat	0 g
Calories	200	Cholesterol	5 mg
Protein	5 g	Phosphorus	138 mg
Carbohydrates	3 g	Potassium	133 mg
Fiber	<1 g	Sodium	130 mg

DIABETIC EXCHANGES
• • • • • •
.22 meat (very lean)
.5 meat (medium fat)
.3 vegetable
3.28 fats

FOR:

- DASH Diet
- Diabetes Diet
- Dialysis Diet
- Heart Health Diet
- Kidney Stone
  Reduction Diet
- Low-Protein Diet
- Post-Transplant Diet
- Vegetarian Diet

ITALIAN DRESSING

Check with your doctor or dietitian to make sure that this recipe is compatible with your current dietary needs and limitations.

YIELD: 14 SERVINGS (ABOUT 1 TABLESPOON EACH)

• • • • • •

$1/4$ cup red wine vinegar

1 tablespoon sugar

2 teaspoons dried oregano

1 teaspoon dried rosemary

$1/8$ teaspoon freshly ground black pepper

1 medium clove garlic, minced

$3/4$ cup extra virgin olive oil

1. Place the vinegar, sugar, oregano, rosemary, pepper, and garlic in a small bowl, and whisk together.

2. Gradually whisk the olive oil into the vinegar mixture.

3. Use to dress green salads. Store any leftover dressing in a covered glass container in the refrigerator for up to 5 days. Bring to room temperature and whisk thoroughly before serving.

NUTRITIONAL FACTS PER SERVING			
		Fat	14 g
		Sat Fat	2 g
• • • • •		Trans Fat	0 g
Calories	130	Cholesterol	0 mg
Protein	0 g	Phosphorus	1 mg
Carbohydrates	1 g	Potassium	8 mg
Fiber	0 g	Sodium	0 mg

DIABETIC EXCHANGES
• • • • • •
2.65 fats

FOR:

■ DASH Diet
■ Diabetes Diet
■ Dialysis Diet
■ Heart Health Diet
■ Kidney Stone
   Reduction Diet
■ Low-Protein Diet
■ Post-Transplant Diet
■ Vegetarian Diet

RASPBERRY VINAIGRETTE

Check with your doctor or dietitian to make sure that this recipe is compatible with your current dietary needs and limitations.

YIELD: 5 SERVINGS (ABOUT 2 TABLESPOONS EACH)

• • • • • •

3 tablespoons raspberry vinegar

I tablespoon Dijon mustard

I teaspoon sugar

I teaspoon minced garlic

I teaspoon minced shallot

I teaspoon raspberry purée

$1/_3$ cup extra virgin olive oil

Freshly ground black pepper to taste

1. Place the vinegar, mustard, sugar, garlic, shallot, and raspberry purée in a small bowl, and whisk together.

2. Gradually whisk the olive oil into the vinegar mixture. Add pepper to taste.

3. Use to dress green salads. Store any leftover dressing in a covered glass container in the refrigerator for up to 5 days. Bring to room temperature and whisk thoroughly before serving.

NUTRITIONAL FACTS PER SERVING				
• • • • •		Fat	14 g	
		Sat Fat	2 g	
		Trans Fat	0 g	
Calories	140	Cholesterol	0 mg	
Protein	0 g	Phosphorus	3 mg	
Carbohydrates	3 g	Potassium	24 mg	
Fiber	0 g	Sodium	75 mg	

DIABETIC EXCHANGES
• • • • •
2.83 fat

FOR:
- DASH Diet
- Diabetes Diet
- Dialysis Diet
- Heart Health Diet
- Kidney Stone
  Reduction Diet
- Low-Protein Diet
- Post-Transplant Diet
- Vegetarian Diet

LEMON-HONEY-CAYENNE VINAIGRETTE

Check with your doctor or dietitian to make sure that this recipe is compatible with your current dietary needs and limitations.

YIELD: 15 SERVINGS (ABOUT 2 TABLESPOONS EACH)

. . . . . .

$^1/_2$ cup honey

$^1/_4$ cup fresh lemon juice

2 tablespoons sherry vinegar

$^1/_4$ cup minced shallot

1 clove garlic, minced

$^1/_8$ teaspoon cayenne pepper

$^1/_2$ cup extra virgin olive oil

$^1/_4$ cup fresh basil leaves

1. Place the honey, lemon juice, vinegar, shallot, garlic, and cayenne pepper in a small bowl, and whisk the ingredients together.

2. Gradually whisk the olive oil into the lemon juice mixture.

3. Tear the basil leaves, and stir them into the dressing.

4. Cover the dressing with plastic wrap and chill for at least an hour before using to dress green salads. Store any leftover dressing in the refrigerator for up to 2 days, whisking thoroughly before using.

NUTRITIONAL FACTS PER SERVING			
		Fat	7 g
		Sat Fat	1 g
. . . . .		Trans Fat	0 g
Calories	100	Cholesterol	0 mg
Protein	0 g	Phosphorus	3 mg
Carbohydrates	10 g	Potassium	23 mg
Fiber	0 g	Sodium	0 mg

DIABETIC EXCHANGES
. . . . . .
1.5 fat
.5 carbs

SWEET AND SAVORY SNACKS

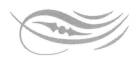

FOR:

- DASH Diet
- Diabetes Diet
- Dialysis Diet
- Heart Health Diet
- Kidney Stone
  Reduction Diet
- Low-Protein Diet
- Post-Transplant Diet
- Vegetarian Diet

ENGLISH MUFFIN PIZZAS

Check with your doctor or dietitian to make sure that this recipe is compatible with your current dietary needs and limitations.

YIELD: 10 SERVINGS

• • • • • •

5 whole wheat English muffins, split in half

2 tablespoons red wine vinegar

2 cloves garlic, minced

1 teaspoon dried oregano

$1/4$ teaspoon freshly ground black pepper

12 leaves fresh basil, divided

20 tomato slices, each about $1/4$ inch thick (4 to 5 medium tomatoes)

1 cup shredded part-skim mozzarella cheese

1. Preheat the broiler of your oven.

2. Line a large baking sheet with aluminum foil, and spray the foil lightly with cooking spray. Arrange the English muffins halves cut-sides-up on the pan, and place under the broiler. Broil for a minute or 2, or until the muffins are lightly toasted.

3. While the muffins are toasting, place the vinegar, garlic, oregano, and pepper in a small bowl, and stir to mix. Chop 2 of the basil leaves and stir them into the vinegar mixture.

4. Top each toasted muffin with 2 slices of tomato. Spread a little of the vinegar mixture over the tomato slices, and sprinkle each pizza with about $1^1/_2$ tablespoons of cheese.

5. Place the pizzas under the preheated broiler and cook for 2 to 3 minutes, or until the cheese is melted. Be careful to avoid burning. Top each pizza with a whole basil leaf and serve immediately.

NUTRITIONAL FACTS PER SERVING			
• • • • •		Fat	3 g
		Sat Fat	1.5 g
		Trans Fat	0 g
Calories	110	Cholesterol	5 mg
Protein	6 g	Phosphorus	164 mg
Carbohydrates	16 g	Potassium	183 mg
Fiber	3 g	Sodium	200 mg

DIABETIC EXCHANGES
• • • • • •
.84 starch
.5 meat (medium fat)
.33 vegetable

SPICY SWEET POTATO CHIPS

Check with your doctor or dietitian to make sure that this recipe is compatible with your current dietary needs and limitations.

YIELD: 10 SERVINGS

• • • • • •

5 sweet potatoes (each about 5 inches long), peeled and sliced $1/_8$-inch thick

$1/_4$ cup canola oil

2 teaspoons chili powder

1 teaspoon garlic powder

$1/_4$ teaspoon paprika

$1/_4$ teaspoon ground cumin

$1/_4$ teaspoon freshly ground black pepper

1. Place the potatoes in a large pot. Cover with room-temperature water and allow to sit for 30 minutes.

2. Drain the potatoes without removing them from the pot, and again cover them with water. Bring the potatoes to a boil and cook for 5 to 10 minutes, or until they are partly cooked, but not yet tender. (They will cook through in the oven.) Drain the potatoes, and pat dry with paper towels or clean kitchen towels.

3. While the potatoes are boiling, line a large baking sheet with aluminum foil, and set aside. Preheat the oven to 400°F.

4. Place the oil and seasonings in a large plastic bag with a zip-type closure. Add the drained and dried potatoes to the bag, seal, and shake until the potatoes are well coated with the seasoned oil.

5. Arrange the potatoes in a single layer on the baking sheet, and place in the preheated oven. Bake for 20 to 25 minutes, or until brown and crisp, flipping the potatoes halfway through the cooking time. Serve immediately.

NUTRITIONAL FACTS PER SERVING			
		Fat	6 g
		Sat Fat	0 g
• • • • •		Trans Fat	0 g
Calories	110	Cholesterol	0 mg
Protein	1 g	Phosphorus	34 mg
Carbohydrates	14 g	Potassium	236 mg
Fiber	2 g	Sodium	45 mg

DIABETIC EXCHANGES
• • • • • •
.7 starch

ZUCCHINI MINI MUFFINS

Check with your doctor or dietitian to make sure that this recipe is compatible with your current dietary needs and limitations.

YIELD: 4 SERVINGS (ABOUT 3 MINI MUFFINS EACH)

• • • • • •

1 medium zucchini

2 large egg whites, lightly beaten

$1/4$ medium onion, minced

$1/4$ cup grated Parmesan cheese

$1/4$ cup plain (unseasoned) bread crumbs

1 clove garlic, minced

1 teaspoon freshly ground black pepper

1 teaspoon dried basil

1. Preheat the oven to 400°F. Spray 12 to 14 cups of a mini muffin pan with nonstick cooking spray, and set aside.

2. Grate the zucchini using a cheese grater. Place the grated zucchini in a paper towel or clean kitchen towel, and wring out any excess water.

3. Place the zucchini and all of the remaining ingredients in a medium-size bowl, and stir to combine.

4. Spoon the zucchini mixture into the mini muffin cups, filling each cup to the top. You should fill 12 to 14 cups.

5. Place the muffin tin in the preheated oven and bake for 20 minutes, or until the muffins are golden brown and set. Serve immediately.

NUTRITIONAL FACTS PER SERVING			
		Fat	2 g
		Sat Fat	1 g
• • • • • •		Trans Fat	0 g
Calories	70	Cholesterol	5 mg
Protein	5 g	Phosphorus	81 mg
Carbohydrates	8 g	Potassium	202 mg
Fiber	1 g	Sodium	180 mg

DIABETIC EXCHANGES
• • • • • •
.33 starch
.25 meat (very lean)
.43 vegetable

FOR:
- DASH Diet
- Diabetes Diet
- Dialysis Diet
- Heart Health Diet
- Kidney Stone Reduction Diet
- Low-Protein Diet
- Post-Transplant Diet
- Vegetarian Diet

ROSEMARY CASHEWS

Check with your doctor or dietitian to make sure that this recipe is compatible with your current dietary needs and limitations.

YIELD: 16 SERVINGS

• • • • • •

1 pound dry-roasted cashews (unsalted) or raw cashews

1 tablespoon olive oil

2 tablespoons chopped fresh rosemary

2 teaspoons brown sugar (not packed)

$^1/_2$ teaspoon cayenne pepper

$^1/_4$ teaspoon salt

1. Preheat the oven to 375°F. Line a large rimmed baking sheet with aluminum foil.

2. Spread the cashews in a single layer on the prepared sheet, and place in the preheated oven. If using dry-roasted cashews, bake for 5 minutes or until the nuts are heated through. If using raw cashews, bake, stirring frequently, for 8 to 10 minutes, or until the nuts are lightly toasted and fragrant.

3. While the cashews are baking, place the remaining ingredients in a large bowl and stir well to combine.

4. Pour the heated cashews into the bowl, and toss well until all the nuts are coated with the seasoned oil. Serve.

NUTRITIONAL FACTS PER SERVING			
• • • • • •		Fat	14 g
		Sat Fat	2.5 g
		Trans Fat	0 g
Calories	170	Cholesterol	0 mg
Protein	4 g	Phosphorus	139 mg
Carbohydrates	10 g	Potassium	163 mg
Fiber	<1 g	Sodium	40 mg

DIABETIC EXCHANGES
• • • • • •
.6 meat (very lean)
3.3 fat

SNACK MIX

Check with your doctor or dietitian to make sure that this recipe is compatible with your current dietary needs and limitations.

YIELD: 12 SERVINGS

•   •   •   •   •   •

3 tablespoons olive oil

1 tablespoon
Worcestershire sauce

$3/_4$ teaspoon Mrs. Dash
seasoning mix (any flavor)
or other no-salt seasoning
blend

$1/_2$ teaspoon garlic powder

$1/_4$ teaspoon onion powder

$3/_4$ cup dry-roasted peanuts
(unsalted)

4 ounces (about 2 cups)
small pretzels (unenriched
flour, unsalted)

3 cups Corn Chex-type
cereal

1. Preheat the oven to 275°F. Line a large rimmed baking sheet with aluminum foil, and set aside.

2. Place the oil, Worcestershire sauce, Mrs. Dash, garlic powder, and onion powder in a small bowl, and stir to mix well.

3. Place the nuts and pretzels in a large bowl, and pour the oil mixture over the top. Stir to coat. Add the cereal, and stir again.

4. Pour the nut mixture onto the prepared pan and spread evenly over the foil. Bake in the preheated oven for 3 hours, stirring occasionally. Cool and serve.

NUTRITIONAL FACTS PER SERVING			
		Fat	8 g
		Sat Fat	1 g
• • • • •		Trans Fat	0 g
Calories	150	Cholesterol	0 mg
Protein	4 g	Phosphorus	67 mg
Carbohydrates	16 g	Potassium	103 mg
Fiber	2 g	Sodium	100 mg

DIABETIC EXCHANGES
• • • • • •
1 starch
.33 meat (very lean)
1.34 fat

FOR:
- DASH Diet
- Diabetes Diet
- Heart Health Diet
- Kidney Stone Reduction Diet
- Low-Protein Diet
- Post-Transplant Diet
- Vegetarian Diet

NOT FOR:
- Dialysis Diet

CRISPY ROASTED CHICKPEAS

Check with your doctor or dietitian to make sure that this recipe is compatible with your current dietary needs and limitations.

YIELD: 8 SERVINGS

• • • • • •

2 (15 ounce) cans no-salt-added chickpeas, rinsed and drained

2 tablespoons olive oil

1 teaspoon chili powder

1 teaspoon ground cumin

$1/_2$ teaspoon cayenne pepper

1. Preheat the oven to 400°F. Line a large rimmed baking sheet with parchment paper, and set aside.

2. Place the rinsed chickpeas in a clean kitchen towel or on paper toweling, and pat dry.

3. Place the chickpeas, olive oil, and spices in a large bowl, and toss until the chickpeas are evenly coated.

4. Spread the chickpeas in an even layer on the prepared baking sheet, and bake in the preheated oven, shaking occasionally, for 30 to 40 minutes, or until crisp. Serve immediately, or allow to cool, place in an airtight container, and store in a cool, dry place for up to three days.

NUTRITIONAL FACTS PER SERVING*			
• • • • •		Fat	4.5 g
		Sat Fat	0 g
		Trans Fat	0 g
Calories	140	Cholesterol	0 mg
Protein	6 g	Phosphorus	83 mg
Carbohydrates	19 g	Potassium	218 mg
Fiber	4 g	Sodium	30 mg

DIABETIC EXCHANGES
• • • • • •
1.33 starch
.66 fat

*Note that Crispy Roasted Chickpeas can be made with different herbs and spices, but this will affect the Nutritional Facts. Check the nutrient counts of any substitute ingredients online. To keep the sodium count down, avoid using salt and blends that contain salt.

FOR:
- DASH Diet
- Diabetes Diet
- Dialysis Diet
- Heart Health Diet
- Kidney Stone
  Reduction Diet
- Low-Protein Diet
- Post-Transplant Diet
- Vegetarian Diet

FRUIT PIZZA

Check with your doctor or dietitian to make sure that this recipe is compatible with your current dietary needs and limitations.

YIELD: I SERVING

• • • • • •

One 3-inch rice cake
(plain or flavored)

I tablespoon plain
whipped cream cheese

$1/4$ cup fresh berries
(blackberries, blueberries,
raspberries, or sliced
strawberries)

1. Spread the cream cheese evenly over the rice cake.

2. Arrange the berries over the cream cheese, pressing lightly to make the berries stick to the "pizza." Serve.

NUTRITIONAL FACTS PER SERVING			
		Fat	2.5 g
		Sat Fat	1.5 g
• • • • •		Trans Fat	0 g
Calories	120	Cholesterol	5 mg
Protein	2 g	Phosphorus	14 mg
Carbohydrates	21 g	Potassium	105 mg
Fiber	1 g	Sodium	100 mg

DIABETIC EXCHANGES
• • • • • •
.88 starch
.34 fruit
.45 fat

FOR:
- DASH Diet
- Diabetes Diet
- Dialysis Diet
- Heart Health Diet
- Low-Protein Diet
- Post-Transplant Diet
- Vegetarian Diet

NOT FOR:
- Kidney Stone Reduction Diet

PEANUT BUTTER BANANA ROLL-UPS

Check with your doctor or dietitian to make sure that this recipe is compatible with your current dietary needs and limitations.

YIELD: 4 SERVINGS

• • • • • •

Two 7- to 8-inch flour tortillas

2 tablespoons natural smooth peanut butter

1 peeled banana, about 8 inches long, halved lengthwise

1. Arrange the tortillas on a flat surface and spread one tablespoon of peanut butter evenly over each of them.

2. Place a banana half on one edge of each tortilla and roll up. Cut each roll-up in half crosswise, and serve immediately.

NUTRITIONAL FACTS PER SERVING		Fat	6 g
		Sat Fat	1 g
• • • • •		Trans Fat	0 g
Calories	150	Cholesterol	0 mg
Protein	4 g	Phosphorus	51 mg
Carbohydrates	21 g	Potassium	157 mg
Fiber	2 g	Sodium	200 mg

DIABETIC EXCHANGES
• • • • • •
1 starch
.5 fruit
.25 meat (lean)
.75 fat

DESSERTS
AND SWEET
TREATS

FOR:

■ DASH Diet
■ Diabetes Diet
■ Dialysis Diet
■ Heart Health Diet
■ Kidney Stone
   Reduction Diet
■ Low-Protein Diet
■ Post-Transplant Diet
■ ~~Vegetarian Diet~~

MERINGUE BITES

Check with your doctor or dietitian to make sure that this recipe is compatible with your current dietary needs and limitations.

YIELD: 40 COOKIES

• • • • • •

4 egg whites

$\frac{1}{4}$ teaspoon cream
of tartar

I teaspoon vanilla extract

$\frac{2}{3}$ cup sugar

1. Preheat the oven to 250° F. Line 2 large baking sheets with parchment paper.

2. Place the egg whites, cream of tartar, and vanilla extract in a large bowl, and beat with an electric mixer at high speed until the mixture is foamy. Add the sugar 1 tablespoon at a time, continuing to beat until the sugar dissolves and the mixture forms stiff peaks.

3. Spoon heaping tablespoons of the meringue onto the prepared baking sheets. Bake for 1 hour and 15 minutes, reducing the oven temperature to 225°F if the cookies begin to brown. Turn the oven off and allow the meringues to cool and dry in the closed oven with the oven light on for 8 hours or overnight. Carefully remove the meringues from the parchment and transfer to an airtight container. In a well-sealed container, the cookies should remain crisp for several days.

NUTRITIONAL FACTS PER COOKIE			
		Fat	0 g
		Sat Fat	0 g
• • • • •		Trans Fat	0 g
Calories	15	Cholesterol	0 mg
Protein	0 g	Phosphorus	0 mg
Carbohydrates	3 g	Potassium	7 mg
Fiber	0 g	Sodium	5 mg

DIABETIC EXCHANGES
• • • • • •
.24 other carbs

FOR:
- DASH Diet
- Diabetes Diet
- Dialysis Diet
- Heart Health Diet
- Kidney Stone
  Reduction Diet
- Low-Protein Diet
- Post-Transplant Diet
- Vegetarian Diet

MANGO SORBET

Check with your doctor or dietitian to make sure that this recipe is compatible with your current dietary needs and limitations

YIELD: 12 SERVINGS

• • • • • •

1 cup sugar

$^3/_4$ cup water

4 cups fresh mango chunks (about 4 mangos, peeled, pitted, and cubed)

3 tablespoons fresh lime juice

1. Place the sugar and water in a small saucepan. Cook over low heat, stirring often, until the sugar has dissolved and the syrup is clear. Set the syrup aside to cool to room temperature.

2. Place the cooled syrup, mango chunks, and lime juice in a blender or food processor, and blend for 30 seconds or until completely smooth.

3. Transfer the mango mixture to a bowl, cover with plastic wrap, and place in the refrigerator until cold.

4. Stir the chilled mango mixture. Then transfer it to an ice cream maker and freeze according to the manufacturer's instructions. When finished, the sorbet will be soft. If you want a firmer dessert, transfer it to a freezer-safe container and place in the freezer for 2 hours before serving.

NUTRITIONAL FACTS PER SERVING			
		Fat	0 g
		Sat Fat	0 g
• • • • •		Trans Fat	0 g
Calories	90	Cholesterol	0 mg
Protein	0 g	Phosphorus	6 mg
Carbohydrates	23 g	Potassium	68 mg
Fiber	<1 g	Sodium	0 mg

DIABETIC EXCHANGES
• • • • • •
.5 fruit
1 other carbs

FOR:

- DASH Diet
- Diabetes Diet
- Dialysis Diet
- Heart Health Diet
- Kidney Stone Reduction Diet
- Low-Protein Diet
- Post-Transplant Diet
- Vegetarian Diet

STRAWBERRY GRANITA

Check with your doctor or dietitian to make sure that this recipe is compatible with your current dietary needs and limitations.

YIELD: 6 SERVINGS

• • • • • •

1 pound ripe strawberries, hulled and sliced (about 3 1/2 cups)

2 tablespoons sugar

1 cup cranberry juice drink

6 tablespoons whipped cream (for garnish)

6 sliced strawberries or whole raspberries (for garnish)

1. Place the strawberries and the sugar in a bowl, and toss to mix. Cover and allow to sit at room temperature for about 1 hour.

2. Transfer the strawberry mixture to a food processor or blender. Add the cranberry drink and process into a chunky purée.

3. Transfer the purée to a shallow dish or tray and place in the freezer for 30 minutes. Using a fork, scrape the frozen edges into the liquid center. Return the dish to the freezer, freeze for another 30 minutes, and again scrape the edges into the center. Repeat this process about 3 more times or until the mixture is fluffy with soft ice crystals.

4. Serve the granita in dessert cups or short-stemmed glasses, garnishing each serving with a tablespoon of whipped cream and a strawberry or raspberry.

NUTRITIONAL FACTS PER SERVING			
• • • • • •		Fat	1 g
		Sat Fat	.5 g
		Trans Fat	0 g
Calories	70	Cholesterol	<5 mg
Protein	<1 g	Phosphorus	24 mg
Carbohydrates	14 g	Potassium	166 mg
Fiber	2 g	Sodium	5 mg

DIABETIC EXCHANGES
• • • • •
.64 fruit
.2 fat
.31 other carbs

FOR:

- DASH Diet
- Diabetes Diet
- Dialysis Diet
- Heart Health Diet
- Kidney Stone Reduction Diet
- Low-Protein Diet
- Post-Transplant Diet
- Vegetarian Diet

RICE PUDDING WITH RAISINS

Check with your doctor or dietitian to make sure that this recipe is compatible with your current dietary needs and limitations

YIELD: 12 SERVINGS

• • • • • •

1 cup white short-grain rice, such as arborio

1 quart rice milk, divided

$1/8$ teaspoon salt

1 teaspoon ground cinnamon

$1/4$ cup pure maple syrup

$1/3$ cup seedless raisins (do not pack)

$1/8$ teaspoon ground cinnamon or nutmeg (for garnish)

1. Place the rice in a strainer, and rinse under cold running water. Transfer the rice to a heavy medium-size saucepan, and stir in 3 cups of the rice milk, the salt, and 1 teaspoon of cinnamon.

2. Bring the rice mixture to a boil over medium-high heat, stirring often to prevent the rice from sticking and the milk from boiling over. Reduce the heat to a gentle simmer and cook, stirring occasionally, for 20 minutes.

3. Add the maple syrup to the rice mixture and cook, stirring often, for about 30 minutes, or until the rice has cooked through and absorbed most of the milk. If the rice starts getting dry during cooking, stir in some of the reserved rice milk.

4. Stir the raisins into the pudding. Serve warm or chilled with a sprinkling of cinnamon or nutmeg.

NUTRITIONAL FACTS PER SERVING			
		Fat	1 g
		Sat Fat	0 g
• • • • •		Trans Fat	0 g
Calories	120	Cholesterol	0 mg
Protein	1 g	Phosphorus	52 mg
Carbohydrates	26 g	Potassium	75 mg
Fiber	<1 g	Sodium	70 mg

DIABETIC EXCHANGES

• • • • • •

.75 starch

.2 fruit

0 fat

.3 other carbs

OLD-FASHIONED BAKED CINNAMON APPLES

Check with your doctor or dietitian to make sure that this recipe is compatible with your current dietary needs and limitations.

YIELD: 6 SERVINGS

6 small tart apples, such as Jonathan or McIntosh

2 cups water

2 teaspoons ground cinnamon

1 1/2 teaspoons vanilla extract

2 tablespoons light brown sugar (for garnish)

1. Preheat the oven to 350°F.

2. Core each apple and remove a 1/2-inch band of peel along the top. Arrange the apples in a 9 x 9-inch baking pan. Set aside.

3. Place the water and cinnamon in a saucepan, and bring to a boil. Stir in the vanilla extract, and pour the mixture over the apples.

4. Place the dish containing the apples in the oven and bake for about 1 hour, or until the apples are easily pierced with a fork. During baking, baste the apples several times with the liquid.

5. Remove the apples from the oven and allow them to cool in the sauce. Serve warm or chilled, topped with some of the sauce and a sprinkling of brown sugar.

NUTRITIONAL FACTS PER SERVING			
Calories	90	Fat	0 g
Protein	0 g	Sat Fat	0 g
Carbohydrates	24 g	Trans Fat	0 g
Fiber	4 g	Cholesterol	0 mg
		Phosphorus	17 mg
		Potassium	168 mg
		Sodium	0 mg

DIABETIC EXCHANGES
1.3 fruit
.41 other carbs

FOR:
- DASH Diet
- Diabetes Diet
- Dialysis Diet
- Heart Health Diet
- Kidney Stone Reduction Diet
- Low-Protein Diet
- Post-Transplant Diet
- Vegetarian Diet

GRILLED MAPLE-AND-SPICE PINEAPPLE

Check with your doctor or dietitian to make sure that this recipe is compatible with your current dietary needs and limitations

YIELD: 4 SERVINGS (2 SLICES EACH)

• • • • • •

1 ripe pineapple, peeled and cut into $1/2$-inch slices

Basting Sauce

2 tablespoons pure maple syrup

1 tablespoon fresh lemon juice

1 teaspoon olive oil

1 teaspoon ground cinnamon

$1/2$ teaspoon ground cloves

1. To make the basting sauce, place all of the sauce ingredients in a small bowl, and whisk to combine well. Set aside.

2. Preheat a gas grill to high, prepare a hot charcoal grill, or preheat an oven broiler to high. Lightly coat the grill or rack with nonstick cooking spray, and place it 4 to 6 inches from the heat source.

3. Lightly brush both sides of the pineapple slices with the prepared basting sauce. Grill the first side for 3 to 5 minutes, or until you have grill marks. Baste the top of the slices once more with the remaining sauce, turn the slices over, and continue to grill for 3 to 5 minutes, or until the fruit is golden on the outside and tender when pierced with a fork. Serve warm.

NUTRITIONAL FACTS PER SERVING			
		Fat	1.5 g
		Sat Fat	0 g
• • • • • •		Trans Fat	0 g
Calories	100	Cholesterol	0 mg
Protein	<1 g	Phosphorus	10 mg
Carbohydrates	23 g	Potassium	159 mg
Fiber	2 g	Sodium	0 mg

DIABETIC EXCHANGES
• • • • • •
1 fruit
.22 fat
.5 other carbs

FOR:
- DASH Diet
- Diabetes Diet
- Dialysis Diet
- Heart Health Diet
- Kidney Stone Reduction Diet
- Low-Protein Diet
- Post-Transplant Diet
- Vegetarian Diet

CRANBERRY OATMEAL COOKIES

Check with your doctor or dietitian to make sure that this recipe is compatible with your current dietary needs and limitations.

YIELD: 24 COOKIES

• • • • •

1¼ cups uncooked old-fashioned oats (cook in 5 minutes)

¾ cup unbleached all-purpose flour

¾ teaspoon ground cinnamon

½ teaspoon baking soda

¾ cup lightly packed brown sugar

½ cup unsweetened applesauce

2 large egg whites

1 teaspoon vanilla extract

¾ cup sweetened dried cranberries

1. Preheat the oven to 350°F. Line 2 large cookie sheets with aluminum foil or parchment, spray with nonstick cooking spray, and set aside.

2. Place the oats, flour, cinnamon, and baking soda in a large bowl, and mix with a whisk until well blended. Set aside.

3. Place the brown sugar and applesauce in a large bowl, and use a fork or hand mixer to combine. Beat or stir in the egg whites and vanilla extract.

4. Add the oat mixture to the applesauce mixture, and stir until blended. Do not over-stir. Gently stir in the cranberries.

5. Drop the dough by rounded tablespoons onto the prepared cookie sheets, spacing the cookies about 1 inch apart.

6. Bake for 10 to 12 minutes, or until the edges are lightly browned and the cookies bounce back when lightly tapped on top. Cool on the sheets for at least 5 minutes before transferring the cookies to a rack to cool completely. Once cool, the cookies can be stored in an airtight glass container for 3 to 4 days.

NUTRITIONAL FACTS PER COOKIE			
• • • • •		Fat	0 g
		Sat Fat	0 g
		Trans Fat	0 g
Calories	60	Cholesterol	0 mg
Protein	<1 g	Phosphorus	5 mg
Carbohydrates	14 g	Potassium	28 mg
Fiber	0 g	Sodium	35 mg

DIABETIC EXCHANGES
• • • • • •
.16 starch
.26 fruit
.5 other carbs

Conclusion

Kidney disease is indeed a chronic condition. However, its course can be controlled with the help of diet, medication, and lifestyle changes. As often stated in this book, the management of CKD has many aspects, and while the best outcome requires the expertise of your healthcare team, it also depends on you. Fortunately, there are a number of steps you can take to slow or even stop the progression of your disease, manage your symptoms, improve your overall well-being, and feel better both physically and emotionally.

This book provides the basics you need to understand and follow the food plan provided by your healthcare team, but to have the best long-term outcome, you must remain proactive. Continue to learn all you can about CKD by reading the literature your team provides and by jotting down questions to ask at each office visit. Browse the websites of the organizations listed in the Resources section of this book (see page 186), and seek out books such as this one, which provides important information and can serve as a ready reference throughout your treatment. Make it a point to ask for any assistance you may need. Whether you are looking for an elusive fact, moral support, or help in sticking to dietary or lifestyle changes, the members of your treatment team can point you in the right direction.

Needless to say, you must be vigilant about following your kidney diet, but since CKD is ever-changing, realize that your treatment plan—including your food plan—will also change. Review your lab test results with your doctor to better understand why particular nutrients must be limited or dietary changes made. Communicate with your dietitian about the best ways for you to restrict targeted substances but still achieve good nutrition. Keep a food diary that your healthcare team can analyze if your test results should change. Seek advice the moment you need it, and speak truthfully about any physical or emotional issues you may be struggling with. Finally, take every possible step you can to improve your fitness and nurture your overall health. The sense of control you will gain over your condition will be worth every bit of effort.

It is my hope that you have found *The Doctor's Kidney Diets* to be invaluable as you learn about CKD and discover how diet plays a crucial role in its management. Always feel free to contact me with questions, comments, or suggestions for future editions. You can reach me at drskidneydiet@gmail.com or, if you prefer, send a letter c/o Square One Publishers, 115 Herricks Road, Garden City Park, NY 11040.

As you now know, preserving kidney function in the face of CKD is a lifelong undertaking that involves the efforts of numerous people. Having read this book, you are better prepared to adopt the mindset and habits that are critical to becoming a knowledgeable, effective participant in your own treatment plan. As you continue the journey that is CKD management, I wish you, your family, and your healthcare team all the best.

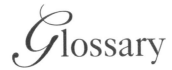

Glossary

Occasionally, this book uses terms that are common in the treatment of kidney disease and associated disorders but may not be completely familiar to you. You may also hear these terms when working with doctors and other healthcare professionals. To help you more easily understand CKD literature and participate in discussions with your healthcare team, definitions are provided below for words that are often used by those who diagnose and treat chronic kidney disease. All terms that appear in *italic type* within the definitions are also defined within the glossary.

acid-base balance. The body's balance between levels of acidity and alkalinity. Healthy *kidneys* help maintain this balance by excreting excess acids and controlling the level of an alkalizing substance called *bicarbonate.*

acid-base homeostasis. See *acid-base balance.*

acute kidney injury (AKI). A type of kidney damage that occurs suddenly due to infection, injury, *glomerulonephritis*, surgery, the ingestion of poison, dehydration, or a severe reaction to a medication or the contrast dye used in imaging procedures.

albumin. The main protein found in human blood.

albuminuria. An abnormally high amount of the protein called *albu-*

min in the urine. Albuminuria is most often a sign of kidney disease, which allows protein to leak out of the blood into the urine.

anemia. A deficiency of red blood cells, the oxygen-carrying components of the blood. People with kidney disease often have anemia because impaired *kidneys* are not able to make a sufficient amount of *erythropoietin,* a hormone that stimulates the bone marrow to produce red blood cells.

antidiuretic hormone (ADH). A hormone that responds to low blood volume by signaling the *kidneys* to reduce and concentrate the urine, thereby keeping water in the blood.

arrhythmia. An irregular heartbeat.

atherosclerosis. A condition in which the arteries are so clogged with plaque—an accumulation of *cholesterol, fat,* and other substances— that blood flow is restricted.

bicarbonate. A very strong base, secreted by the stomach and intestines, that helps keeps the *pH* of the blood from becoming too acidic. One of the ways in which *kidneys* help control pH is by regulating the amount of bicarbonate that is present.

bisphenol A (BPA). An industrial chemical with toxic properties that is used to make plastic water bottles, the coating of food and beverage cans, and other food containers. Under some circumstances, BPA can leach into foods, posing a health risk.

bladder. The organ of the *urinary system* that collects urine excreted by the *kidneys* and stores it prior to its release from the body through urination.

blood glucose. See *blood sugar.*

blood pressure. The pressure exerted by the blood against the blood vessels as the heart pumps. *High blood pressure,* also called hypertension, is a common cause of kidney disease.

blood sugar. Also called blood glucose, the concentration of the sugar *glucose* in the blood, measured in milligrams of glucose per 100 milliliters of blood. High blood sugar levels, known as *hyperglycemia,* occur when the body has too little *insulin* or when it is unable to use insulin properly. See also *diabetes.*

blood urea nitrogen (BUN) test. A test that measures the amount of nitrogen in the blood resulting from the waste product *urea.* This test is often used along with *creatinine* tests to help determine kidney function.

body mass index (BMI). A measure of body fat based on a person's height and weight. The BMI is used as an indicator of risk for a number of disorders, including heart and kidney disease.

body pH. See *acid-base balance.*

BUN test. See *blood urea nitrogen test.*

calcitriol. Also known as vitamin D_3, an active form of *vitamin D* that enables the body to absorb *calcium* from the gut. Healthy *kidneys* are able to produce calcitriol from vitamin D that is received from food and sunlight. When kidney function is impaired, calcitriol can be taken in supplement form.

calcium. A mineral needed for bone health and for the proper function of the heart, muscles, and nerves. Problems caused by *chronic kidney disease* can prevent calcium from being properly used by the body and cause it to be deposited in the blood vessels, where it contributes to *cardiovascular disease.*

carbohydrate counting. A meal-planning technique, used by diabetics, that helps manage blood glucose levels by tracking the amount of *carbohydrates* consumed.

carbohydrates. One of the three main types of nutrients, the others being *protein* and *fat.* The most important source of energy for the body, carbohydrates are defined chemically as compounds of carbon, hydrogen, and oxygen. They include sugars, starches, and fiber.

cardiovascular disease (CVD). A range of conditions that involve the heart or blood vessels. CVD—especially *high blood pressure* and *atherosclerosis*—is common in people with *chronic kidney disease.*

cholesterol. A waxy substance that is necessary for the building and maintaining of the body's cells and for making bile acids, hormones, vitamin D, and other essential chemicals. When too much cholesterol is consumed, however, it can form deposits in blood vessels that can lead to *cardiovascular disease.* See also *high-density lipoprotein cholesterol* and *low-density lipoprotein cholesterol.*

chronic inflammation. A persistent inflammatory condition that slowly and continuously attacks and damages the internal organs. Different from acute inflammation, which is a normal response to injury or illness, chronic inflammation has been increasingly identified as an underlying cause of many illnesses, including kidney disease, heart disease, *diabetes,* and cancer.

chronic kidney disease (CKD). A gradual loss of *kidney* function that is usually permanent. The most common form of kidney disease, CKD is defined in terms of five stages, with Stage 1 being the least severe and Stage 5 indicating kidney failure, or *end-stage renal disease.*

congenital kidney disease. Structural problems or blockages of the *kidney* that are present at birth, as well as hereditary kidney disorders.

creatinine. A normal waste product of muscle metabolism that passes through the *kidneys* and, when kidneys are healthy, is filtered out and eliminated through the urine. This substance is measured to determine kidney function and to calculate eGFR, or *estimated glomerular filtration rate.*

DASH diet. An eating plan designed to help prevent or treat *high blood pressure* (hypertension), and can also slow the progression of early stage *chronic kidney disease* (CKD). DASH is short for Dietary Approaches to Stop Hypertension.

diabetes. A group of disorders characterized by higher-than-normal levels of *glucose* (sugar) in the blood. The three main types of diabetes include gestational diabetes, which occurs in expectant women and usually disappears at the pregnancy's end; type 1 diabetes, in which the *blood sugar* level is high because the body produces little or no *insulin,* the hormone that permits glucose to be absorbed and used by the cells; and type 2 diabetes, in which the body's cells are unable to use insulin properly.

dialysis. The process of filtering toxins and excess fluids from the blood, usually through the use of a machine.

edema. Excess fluid trapped in the body's tissues, most often observed as swelling in the arms, hands, legs, ankles, and feet. Edema is a common symptom of *chronic kidney disease.*

electrolytes. Minerals that conduct electrical impulses in the body and are necessary for the regulation of fluids, the generation of energy, and many other biochemical reactions. The body's major electrolytes include *bicarbonate, calcium,* chloride, *magnesium, phosphorus, potassium,* and *sodium.*

end-stage renal disease (ESRD). Stage 5 of *chronic kidney disease,* in which the *kidneys* fail to function completely or almost completely, requiring *dialysis* or kidney transplant. This condition is also called kidney failure, renal failure, and end-stage kidney disease.

erythropoietin (EPO). A hormone released by the *kidneys* that stimulates the bone marrow to create more red blood cells.

estimated glomerular filtration rate (eGFR). A measure of how efficiently the *kidneys* are able to filter toxins and excess fluids from the blood, and therefore, how well they are functioning. The eGFR is based on blood tests that calculate the level of *creatinine* (a waste product) in the blood.

fats. One of the three main types of nutrients, the others being *carbohydrates* and *protein.* Fats are a major source of energy in the diet, help the body absorb certain nutrients, and perform other vital functions. But because of their high calorie content, when fats are eaten in excess, they can lead to obesity, and some fats—*saturated fats* and *trans fats*—can increase the risk of *cardiovascular disease.*

fiber. A type of *carbohydrate* that passes through the body undigested. Soluble fiber dissolves in water and can help lower *glucose* levels by slowing digestion, and thereby slowing the release of *glucose* into the blood. It may also help to regulate *cholesterol.* Insoluble fiber, which does not dissolve in water, adds bulk to waste, helping it move more quickly through the digestive system.

glomerulonephritis (GN). Also called nephritis, a kidney disorder caused by damage to or scarring of the *glomeruli*—the *kidneys'* tiny filtering units.

glomerulus (*pl.* glomeruli). Found within the *nephron* (a structure within the *kidneys*), a network of tiny blood vessels that remove wastes and toxins from the blood.

glucose. A simple sugar that is the primary source of energy for the human body. Glucose is obtained from *carbohydrates*—starches and sugars consumed in the form of grains, legumes, fruits, and vegetables. When a disorder such as *diabetes* causes high levels of glucose to remain in the blood, rather than being absorbed and used by the cells, the glucose damages the filtering units of the *kidneys,* impairing the organs' ability to remove wastes and excess water from the blood.

glycemic index (GI). A measure of the impact a *carbohydrate*-containing food has on *blood sugar* levels. Items with a high GI raise blood glucose more than foods with a low or medium GI.

gout. A form of arthritis characterized by severe periods of pain, redness, swelling, and tenderness in the joints, often at the base of the big toe. The incidence of gout is associated with higher-than normal levels of *uric acid,* which can form sharp, painful crystals in the joints and surrounding tissues.

high blood pressure. Also called hypertension, a condition in which the force of blood flowing against blood vessel walls is high enough to cause health problems. Over time, high blood pressure can stretch and damage blood vessels and create serious heart and kidney disorders, as well as stroke.

high-density lipoprotein (HDL) cholesterol. A type of *cholesterol,* often referred to as "good" cholesterol, that carries excess cholesterol away from the body's cells to the liver for removal.

hyperglycemia. Also called high blood glucose, a condition that occurs when the body produces too little of the hormone *insulin* or is unable to use insulin properly, resulting in higher-than-normal levels of *glucose* (sugar) in the blood. See also *diabetes.*

hypertension. See *high blood pressure.*

hyperuricemia. An abnormally high blood level of *uric acid.* Healthy *kidneys* remove excess uric acid from the body, but damaged kidneys are unable to eliminate the acid, allowing it to build up in the blood. When these high levels continue for a long time, painful crystals may form in the joints, causing *gout.*

insoluble fiber. A type of *fiber* that does not dissolve in water. Insoluble fiber adds bulk to waste, helping it move more quickly through the digestive system. Foods high in insoluble fiber include whole grains, seeds, nuts, fruits, and vegetables.

insulin. A hormone, made by the pancreas, that enables the cells of the body to absorb *glucose* (a form of sugar) from the blood and use it for energy. Insulin helps balance *blood sugar* levels and keeps them in a normal range. When the body doesn't produce sufficient insulin or the cells are resistant to the effects of insulin, *diabetes*—a disorder characterized by higher-than-normal levels of glucose (sugar) in the blood—results.

kidney failure. See *end-stage renal disease.*

kidney stones. Small, hard deposits of minerals that form in the *kidneys*. The four major types of stones include calcium stones, the most common; uric acid stones; struvite stones, which are related to certain infections; and cystine stones, which are due to a genetic disorder. People with *chronic kidney disease* have an increased risk of developing this disorder.

kidney vitamins. See *renal vitamins.*

kidneys. The bean-shaped organs of the *urinary system* whose chief function is to remove waste products, excess minerals, and excess fluids from the body. The kidneys also balance the body's fluids, help regulate blood pressure, maintain the body's *acid-base balance,* protect bone health, and control the production of red blood cells.

lipid panel. Also called a lipid profile, a group of tests that measure blood levels of *cholesterol (high-density lipoproteins* and *low-density lipoproteins)* and *triglycerides,* and thereby help healthcare professionals assess the risk of *cardiovascular disease.*

lipids. *Fats*—including *cholesterol* and *triglycerides*—that serve important functions in the body, including the storage of fuel and the building and maintaining of cells. When present in excess, however, lipids increase the risk of *cardiovascular disease.*

lipoproteins. Molecules made of *proteins* and *fats* that carry *cholesterol* and similar substances throughout the blood. See *high-density lipoprotein cholesterol* and *low-density lipoprotein cholesterol.*

low-density lipoprotein (LDL) cholesterol. A type of *cholesterol*, often referred to as "bad" cholesterol, that carries cholesterol to the body's cells. LDL cholesterol can collect in the walls of the blood vessels, causing *atherosclerosis*.

magnesium. A mineral needed to maintain heart rhythm, aid normal nerve and muscle function, keep bones strong, support a healthy immune system, and help regulate *blood sugar* levels and *blood pressure*. Blood levels of magnesium are normally controlled by the *kidneys*, but kidney disease can result in magnesium levels that are too high or too low, leading to serious health problems.

medical nutrition therapy (MNT). An individualized dietary plan, created and monitored by a dietitian, that is designed to treat a specific medical condition and its symptoms.

monounsaturated fats. A type of *unsaturated fat* that can improve blood cholesterol levels and decrease the risk of *cardiovascular disease*. Foods high in monounsaturated fats include olive oil, canola oil, peanut oil, safflower oil, and sesame oil, as well as a number of nuts and seeds.

nephritis. See *glomerulonephritis*.

nephrologist. A medical doctor who specializes in the diagnosis and management of kidney disease.

nephron. The functional unit of the kidney that removes waste products and excess water from the blood and forms urine.

omega-3 fatty acids. A type of *polyunsaturated fat* that can improve blood cholesterol levels and has anticoagulant properties. Foods high in omega-3 fatty acids include flaxseed oil and fatty fish such as salmon and mackerel.

oxalate. A compound naturally present in many foods that can combine with other chemicals and form a type of *kidney stone* known as calcium oxalate kidney stones.

parathyroid hormone (PTH). A hormone, released by the body, that helps regulate the blood's *calcium* and *phosphorus* levels by causing the bones to release calcium into the blood and reducing the amount of calcium eliminated by the kidneys.

pH. A number between 0 and 14 that indicates whether a substance is acid or alkaline (base). A substance with a pH less than 7 is acidic, and a substance with a pH greater than 7 is said to be alkaline. A pH of 7 indicates that the substance is neutral. Healthy *kidneys* help to create a healthy *acid-base balance* in the body.

phosphorus. A mineral needed for bone health and for the body's use of *fats* and *carbohydrates.* Blood levels of phosphorus are normally controlled by the *kidneys,* but when kidney function is impaired, phosphorus levels can rise, leading to bone pain, bone thinning, fractures, and heart disease.

polyunsaturated fats. A type of *unsaturated fat* that can improve blood cholesterol levels and decrease the risk of heart disease. Foods high in polyunsaturated fats include soybean oil, corn oil, and sunflower oil, as well as fatty fish such as herring, mackerel, and salmon.

potassium. A mineral needed for the healthy function of the heart, muscles, and nerves. Blood levels of potassium are normally controlled by the *kidneys,* but when kidney function is impaired, potassium levels can rise, leading to symptoms such as weakness, numbness, and tingling, as well as dangerous changes in heart rhythm.

protein. One of the three main types of nutrients, the others being *carbohydrates* and *fats.* Protein is required for the growth and repair of cells and tissues and to control energy, assist with digestion, and aid in other body functions. Because impaired *kidneys* cannot filter out the potentially toxic byproducts of protein metabolism, people with *chronic kidney disease* often have to restrict protein consumption.

proteinuria. Also called *albuminuria,* an abnormally high amount of *protein* in the urine. Proteinuria is most often a sign of kidney disease, which allows protein to leak out of the blood and into the urine.

pruritis. Intense chronic itching of the skin that is often associated with *uremia.*

PTH. See *parathyroid hormone.*

purines. Substances, found in virtually all foods, that are metabolized by the body into *uric acid.* When uric acid levels become too high, uric acid crystals can form in the joints, leading to *gout*. This is why high-purine foods are often eliminated from the diet as a means of preventing the recurrence of gout.

renal disease. A general term for any condition—including *chronic kidney disease*—in which the kidneys have a lesser ability to filter out waste materials from the blood and perform other necessary functions.

renal system. See *urinary system*.

renal vitamins. Also called kidney vitamins, these are multivitamin supplements specifically designed for people with kidney disease. They are formulated to contain the essential nutrients needed by the CKD patient while avoiding *phosphorus, potassium,* and other nutrients that kidney patients usually must limit.

renin. A *protein* released by the body in response to decreased levels of *sodium* or low *blood pressure*. This results in a chain of events that increase blood pressure.

salt. See *sodium*.

saturated fats. A type of fat that is "saturated" with hydrogen atoms and is solid at room temperature. A diet high in saturated fats has been linked to an increased risk of *cardiovascular disease*. The foods highest in saturated fats include butter, cheese, lard, cream, and fatty cuts of beef, lamb, pork, and poultry.

sodium. A mineral that is important to brain and nerve function and regulates the volume of body fluids. Blood levels of sodium are normally controlled by the *kidneys,* but when kidney function is impaired, sodium is retained by the body, leading to conditions such as *high blood pressure* and *edema*.

soluble fiber. A type of *fiber* that dissolves in water. Soluble fiber slows digestion, and therefore can help lower *blood sugar* levels by slowing the release of *glucose* into the blood. Foods high in soluble fiber include oatmeal, lentils, nuts, and seeds.

sucrose. A crystalline form of sugar, usually referred to simply as sugar. Commercially, sucrose is usually obtained from sugarcane or sugar beets. A high consumption of this substance can contribute to *diabetes*, obesity, *kidney stones*, and other health disorders.

trans fats. A commercial product that is made by hydrogenating liquid vegetable oils to create a solid fat. Trans fats, the most common of which is partially hydrogenated oils, raise levels of "bad" *low-density lipoprotein cholesterol* and lower levels of "good" *high-density lipoprotein cholesterol*, thereby increasing the risk of *cardiovascular disease.*

triglycerides. A type of fat (*lipid*), found in the blood, that stores unused calories and provides the body with energy. High triglyceride levels are associated with an increased risk of *cardiovascular disease.*

type 1 diabetes. A form of *diabetes* in which the *blood sugar* level is high because the body produces little or no *insulin,* the hormone that enables *glucose* to pass from the bloodstream into the body's cells, where it can be used.

type 2 diabetes. A form of *diabetes* in which the body's cells are unable to properly use *insulin,* the hormone that enables *glucose* to pass from the bloodstream into the body's cells, where it can be used. Type 2 is the most common form of diabetes.

unsaturated fats. A type of dietary *fat,* including both *polyunsaturated fats* and *monounsaturated fats,* that is liquid at room temperature. Most unsaturated fats come from vegetable oils, nuts, and fish. These fats can improve blood cholesterol levels, decreasing the risk of *cardiovascular disease.*

urea. A nitrogen-containing waste product, resulting from the breakdown of dietary *protein,* that is normally filtered out of the blood by the *kidneys* and eliminated through the urine.

uremia. A toxic buildup of waste products, such as *urea* and *creatinine,* that would normally be filtered out of the blood by the *kidneys* and excreted in the urine. A serious complication of kidney disease, uremia causes fluid, *electrolyte,* and hormone imbalances that can result in symptoms such as nausea, vomiting, confusion, agitation, chronic itching (*pruritis*), and heart problems such as irregular heartbeat. Uremia means "urine in blood."

uremic symptoms. The symptoms of *uremia.*

ureters. The two thin tubes that connect the *kidneys* to the *bladder;* part of the *urinary system.*

urethra. The tube that allows urine to pass out of the body.

uric acid. A chemical created when the body metabolizes substances called *purines*, which are found in foods. When *kidneys* are healthy, excess uric acid is removed from the body through the urine. When kidney function is impaired, uric acid accumulates in the body, leading to a variety of disorders, including *gout*, the worsening of *chronic kidney disease*, and *uremia*.

urinalysis. An array of tests performed on a urine sample to detect unwanted substances such as *glucose, protein*, or blood cells.

urinary system. Also called the renal system, a body system that includes the *kidneys, ureters, bladder*, and *urethra*. The purpose of the urinary system is to produce, collect, and eliminate urine from the body.

vegan diet. A dietary plan that does not include any animal products at all, and therefore excludes not only meat but also dairy products, eggs, and honey.

vegetarian diet. A dietary plan that focuses on plant foods—fruits, vegetables, beans, grains, seeds, and nuts—and does not include meat or seafood. Most vegetarians include dairy products and eggs in their diet. Some vegetarians, called pescatarians, also eat fish.

vitamin D. A group of fat-soluble vitamins whose chief function is to aid the body's absorption of *calcium* and maintain normal blood levels of calcium and *phosphorus*. It has been suggested that this vitamin also helps reduce the risk of heart disease, *diabetes,* and cancer. Healthy *kidneys* help transform vitamin D, obtained from exposure to sunlight or diet, into an active form that can be used by the body. When kidney function is impaired, vitamin D deficiency can result, requiring the use of activated vitamin D supplements. See also *calcitriol*.

$\mathcal{R}$esources

As you learn about kidney disease management, there will probably be times when you want additional information about kidney-friendly diets, specific foods and nutrients, laboratory tests, or other aspects of CKD. You may also want to learn more about related conditions such as diabetes and heart disease. The listings below will guide you to solid sources of essential health information. To help you browse more efficiently, the lists have been separated into two categories: books related to kidney disease and kidney diets, and organizations whose websites provide a wealth of information about CKD and associated health problems. Be aware that these listings represent just a few of the many books and organizations that can provide you with information, practical advice, and support. A computer search for topics of interest—"low-potassium foods," for instance—will lead you to further resources.

BOOKS TO INFORM AND ASSIST

Brookhyser-Hogan, Joan. *The Vegetarian Diet for Kidney Disease: Preserving Kidney Function with Plant-Based Eating*. Laguna Beach, CA: Basic Health Publications, 2010.

Written by a registered dietician, this book focuses on vegetarian eating as an effective means of managing kidney disease. Specific information is presented to help you implement or continue a plant-based diet for the benefit of your kidneys.

Brown, Susan E., and Larry Trivieri, Jr. *The Acid-Alkaline Food Guide: A Quick Reference to Foods and Their Effect on pH Levels.* Second Edition. Garden City Park, NY: Square One Publishers, 2013.

This easy-to-use guide focuses on the way foods impact your body's pH level. Information is provided about the effect of foods on the body's acid-alkaline balance, and suggestions are given to help you make healthy food choices. The book also lists thousands of foods and food combinations and their acid-alkaline effects so you can select the foods that are right for you.

Chatham, John. *The DASH Diet for Beginners: Essentials to Get Started.* Berkeley, CA: Rockridge University Press, 2013.

This diet guide discusses the health benefits of the DASH eating plan and presents a list of the diet's top recommended foods. Also included is a seven-day meal plan to jump-start your diet, as well as a collection of forty low-sodium recipes.

Cousins, Norman. *Anatomy of an Illness: As Perceived by the Patient.* New York: W.W. Norton and Company, 2005.

This inspirational classic describes the author's use of laughter, courage, and tenacity to triumph over a life-threatening illness. The book was the first to endorse patients' participation in their own care, and it helped establish the importance of taking charge of one's health.

Hulett, Victoria L., and Jennifer L. Waybright. *Smoothies for Kidney Health.* Garden City Park, NY: Square One Publishers, 2015.

Written by a kidney transplant recipient and her donor daughter, "Smoothies for Kidney Health" explains in detail the connection between certain foods and kidney disease. Eighty smoothie recipes are included to help alleviate CKD symptoms, preserve kidney function, and benefit overall health.

Kolbe, Nina. *Kidney Health Gourmet Diet Guide & Cookbook.* Washington, DC: Nina Kolbe, 2011.

This dietary guide and cookbook was designed for patients diagnosed with CKD but not on dialysis. Written by a renal dietitian, it presents nutritional information and more than 200 recipes that can help prevent progression to end-stage renal disease.

Lieberman, Shari. *Glycemic Index Food Guide: For Weight Loss, Cardiovascular Health, Diabetic Management, and Maximum Energy.* Garden City Park, NY: Square One Publishers, 2006.

Written by a leading nutritionist, this book provides answers to commonly asked questions about carbohydrates, blood glucose, and the glycemic index. Included are the glycemic index and glycemic load of hundreds of foods and beverages, including raw foods, cooked foods, and many combination and prepared foods.

Snyder, Mariza, Lauren Clum, and Anna V. Zulaica. *The DASH Diet Cookbook: Quick and Delicious Recipes for Losing Weight, Preventing Diabetes, and Lowering Blood Pressure.* Berkeley, CA: Ulysses Press, 2012.

This helpful cookbook contains 140 easy-to-make recipes that simplify the DASH diet. Complete nutritional information is provided so that you can choose the dishes that match your dietary needs and limitations.

Snyder, Rich. *What You Must Know About Dialysis: The Secrets to Surviving and Thriving on Dialysis.* Garden City Park, NY: Square One Publishers, 2013.

This complete guide to dialysis not only provides answers to common questions about the process, but also offers practical advice and strategies as well as complementary options that can help you deal successfully with the many aspects of your treatment plan. Crucial information is provided on natural supplements, lifestyle changes, nutrition, and effective coping tactics.

Snyder, Rich. *What You Must Know About Kidney Disease: A Practical Guide to Using Conventional and Complementary Treatments.* Garden City Park, NY: Square One Publishers, 2010.

With the goal of providing the information needed to cope with kidney problems, this book begins by offering an overview of kidney structure and function. Part Two then examines kidney disorders and their conventional treatment, and Part Three explores a range of effective complementary therapies, from acupuncture and nutritional supplementation to osteopathic manipulation.

Warshaw, Hope S., and Karmeen Kulkarni. *The Complete Guide to Carb Counting.* Third Edition. Alexandria, VA: American Diabetes Association, 2011.

Created by the American Diabetes Association, this book gives you the information and tools you need to use carbohydrate counting to control blood sugar. Included are the carb counts of everyday foods as well as a guide to counting carbs using food labels and restaurant menus.

ORGANIZATIONS AND WEBSITES

American Association of Kidney Patients (AAKP)
2701 North Rocky Point Drive, Suite 150
Tampa, FL 33607
Phone: 800-749-2257
Website: www.aakp.org
This nonprofit organization strives to improve the lives of people with CKD as well as those who are undergoing dialysis or considering a kidney transplant. The AAKP website offers extensive information about all aspects of kidney disease, along with links to booklets, charts, and useful tools for learning about and managing kidney disease.

American Diabetes Association (ADA)
1701 North Beauregard Street
Alexandria, VA 22311
Phone: 800-342-2383
Website: www.diabetes.org
The ADA provides objective information on all aspects of diabetes, including prevention, diagnosis, medical treatment and care, making healthy food choices, and getting and staying fit. Click on the website's "Food & Fitness" link for valuable information on nutrition, meal-planning, dining out, weight loss, and fitness.

American Heart Association (AHA)
7272 Greenville Avenue
Dallas, TX 75231
Phone: 800-242-8721
Website: www.heart.org
In addition to providing information about various types of heart disease, the American Heart Association website offers information on good nutrition—including healthy cooking tips, recipes, and more—as well as guidance on stress management, weight management, and physical activity.

American Kidney Fund (AKF)
11921 Rockville Pike, Suite 300
Rockville, MD 20852
Phone: 800-638-8299
Website: www.kidneyfund.org
The AKF website provides basic information about kidney function, kidney problems, laboratory tests, kidney-friendly foods, and more. In addition, the AKF offers

grants for people who need assistance meeting the costs of treating kidney failure, with more than 84,000 patients receiving help each year. Patients on dialysis who seek monetary support can get details about the organization from the social worker at their dialysis center.

Davita, Inc.
2000 16th Street
Denver, CO 80202
Phone: 800-244-0680
Website: www.davita.com
The website of this leading dialysis provider presents a wide range of valuable resources for people with CKD, including informative articles about kidney disease and treatment, kidney diet recipes, and links to online discussions. Click on "Food Analyzer" to learn the nutrient content of the foods you eat.

Diabetic Exchange List
Website: http://glycemic.com/DiabeticExchange/The%20Diabetic%20Exchange%20List.pdf
The exchange lists presented on this website are the basis of a meal planning system designed by a committee of the American Diabetes Association and the American Dietetic Association. Although it is intended for people who have diabetes, the exchange system is grounded in the principles of good nutrition, and so can be used by anyone.

EatRight
Website: www.eatright.org/public
Presented by the American Dietetic Association, this website provides helpful nutritional information for people with kidney disease, as well as dietary guidelines, recipes, and a host of tips for planning, shopping, and preparing healthy meals. Click first on "Health," then on "Kidney Disease."

Fresenius Medical Care
920 Winter Street
Waltham, MA 02451
Phone: 800-662-1237
Website: www.freseniusmedicalcare.us/en/home/
This website for later-stage CKD patients and their families provides links to helpful information about the kidneys and kidney disease. Click on "Patients & Families," and choose the topic in which you are interested.

Life Options

c/o Medical Education Institute, Inc.
414 D'Onofrio Drive, Suite 200
Madison, WI 53719
Phone: 800-468-7777
Website: www.lifeoptions.org
This nonprofit program uses research, education, and outreach to improve the lives of people with kidney disease. The Life Options website offers a Kidney Glossary, as well as facts about CKD, patient stories and suggestions, and a Resources page with links for patients and professionals. The site also provides access to "Kidney School," an interactive learning center with sixteen informative modules that can be viewed or listened to online.

National Diabetes Education Program (NDEP)

One Diabetes Way
Bethesda, MD 20814-9692
Phone: 301-496-3583
Website: www.ndep.nih.gov/
This education program is a partnership of the National Institutes of Health, the Centers for Disease Control and Prevention, and more than 200 public and private organizations. The NDEP website presents a wealth of facts and tools for people who have or are at risk of developing diabetes, as well as their families.

National Diabetes Information Clearinghouse (NDIC)

Website: www.niddk.nih.gov/
A joint effort of the National Institute of Diabetes and Digestive and Kidney Diseases (NIDDK) and the National Institutes of Health (NIH), this website presents extensive information about diabetes, including research and statistics, as well as links to drug information, journals, articles, and publications. Also provided is a directory of diabetes organizations and a link through which you can subscribe to an electronic newsletter.

National Institute of Diabetes and Digestive and Kidney Diseases (NIDDK)

9000 Rockville Pike
Bethesda, MD 20892
Phone: 301-496-3583
Website: www.niddk.nih.gov/
NIDDK supports medical research and training while offering educational and outreach programs for patients, their families, healthcare professionals, and the public.

The institute's website contains links to brochures, fact sheets, management tools, and other resources for people with diabetes, kidney disease, and other health conditions.

National Kidney Disease Education Program (NKDEP)
3 Kidney Information Way
Bethesda, MD 20892
Phone: 866-454-3639
Website: www.nkdep.nih.gov/
An initiative of the National Institute of Diabetes and Digestive and Kidney Diseases (NIDDK), the National Institutes of Health (NIH), and the U.S. Department of Health & Human Services (HHS), the NKDEP provides a wealth of information for people who are at risk of developing or already living with kidney disease. Click on "Learn About Kidney Disease" or "Living With Kidney Disease" to find topics of interest.

National Kidney Foundation (NKF)
30 East 33rd Street
New York, NY 10016
Phone: 800-622-9010
Website: www.kidney.org
For DASH diet information:
https://www.kidney.org/atoz/content/Dash_Diet
For information on herbal supplements and CKD:
https://www.kidney.org/atoz/content/herbalsupp
This foundation works to improve the lives of people who have or are at risk of developing kidney disease. The NKF website offers a vast array of important information and sources of assistance. A helpful Search feature can guide you to the subject you want to explore. For detailed information on the DASH diet, use the second link listed above. For lists of herbal supplements that can pose a hazard to people with CKD, click on the third link.

The Nephron Information Center
Website: www.nephron.com/
For nutrient values of food: www.foodvalues.us
Many of this site's offerings are geared toward the medical community, but there are several helpful tools for patients. The homepage features a detailed Search feature complete with drop-down menus to simplify your quest for information. In addition, there are links to a Question/Answer page, kidney blogs, and news articles about kidney disease. For truly complete nutritional information on any food, use the second link listed above.

Partnership for Prescription Assistance (PPA)

Website: www.pparx.org

The PPA is designed to help qualifying patients without prescription drug coverage to get the medication they need—often at little or no cost. The Partnership provides access to more than 475 public and private patient assistance programs, including almost 200 programs offered by pharmaceutical companies.

SELF Nutrition Data

Website: www.nutritiondata.com

This useful site presents information about many topics related to nutrition. Some elements are particularly helpful to kidney patients, including a Search feature that allows you to type in a food name to learn the item's complete nutritional content. You can also create lists of foods that are high or low in a nutrient you have been told to monitor.

Southwest Kidney Institute (SKI)

2149 East Warner Road, Suite 101

Tempe, AZ 85284

Phone: 480-610-6100

Website: www.swkidney.com

This website of a leading nephrology group offers a convenient Search feature through which information and answers can be sought, as well as an Education Center with links to CKD information, articles, and other resources for patients.

The University of Sydney Glycemic Index Database

Website: www.glycemicindex.com/

This website is maintained by the University of Sydney's GI Group, which includes research scientists and dietitians working in the area of glycemic index, health, and nutrition. Type in the name of a food to learn its glycemic index and glycemic load, or click on "About GI" to learn more about this system of selecting foods according to their effect on blood sugar levels.

$\mathcal{A}$ Guide to Foods Low and High in Potassium, Phosphorus, and Sodium

In Chapter 3, you learned that, especially in the later stages of chronic kidney disease, it is often necessary to limit your consumption of those nutrients that your kidneys are no longer able to filter out and eliminate from the body. If you have been told to restrict or steer clear of foods high in potassium, phosphorus, or sodium, you'll find the following lists helpful. Use them to find foods that are relatively low in these minerals as well as to identify foods that are high in these minerals. Just remember that although a wise choice of foods is important, it's just as important to limit portion size, as even a low-potassium (or low-phosphorus) food can provide too much of this nutrient if eaten in large quantities. Be sure to talk to your doctor or dietitian about the foods and serving sizes that are most appropriate for you.

For full discussions of these minerals and CKD, turn to pages 38 to 45. To learn the complete nutritional values of these and other foods, visit the Food Values website of the Nephron Information Center. (See page 189 of the Resources list.)

LOW-POTASSIUM FOOD SOURCES

Apples

Asparagus

Berries

Bread, other than whole grain

Broccoli, raw

Carrots, cooked

Cauliflower

Celery

Cherries

Corn

Cranberries

Cucumbers

Garlic

Grapes

Green beans

Lettuce

Onions

Pasta and noodles, other than whole grain

Peaches

Peppers

Pineapple

Plums

Tangerines

White rice

Yellow summer squash

Zucchini squash

HIGH-POTASSIUM FOODS TO LIMIT OR AVOID

Acorn squash

Apricots

Avocados

Bananas

Beans

Beets

Broccoli, cooked

Brown rice

Brussels sprouts

Carrots, raw, and carrot juice

Chocolate

Clams

Dark leafy greens

Dates

Figs

Kiwi

Lentils

Mangos

Melons

Milk, cheese, yogurt, and other dairy products

Mushrooms

Nectarines

Nuts

Okra

Oranges and orange juice

Peanuts

Pomegranates

Potatoes, white or sweet

Prunes and prune juice

Raisins

Rutabagas

Salt substitutes that contain potassium

Sardines

Soy milk, cheese, and yogurt

Tomatoes and tomato juice

Wheat germ

Whole-grain bread

Whole-grain pasta and noodles

Winter squash

LOW-PHOSPHORUS FOOD SOURCES

Atlantic cod and grouper

Barley, pearled

Bread, other than whole grain

Catsup, salt-free

Corn flakes or crispy rice cereal

Eggs

Farina and hominy grits

Gelatin

Oysters

Pasta and noodles, other than whole grain

Pork, lean

Poultry (skinless), such as chicken, duck, or turkey breast

Sherbet

Shrimp

Soy milk

White rice

HIGH-PHOSPHORUS FOODS TO LIMIT OR AVOID

Beans, including dried, canned, and baked

Beer and ale

Bologna

Bran cereal

Brewer's yeast

Brown rice

Cake

Canned iced tea

Caramels

Chocolate

Chocolate drinks

Crayfish

Dark colas and certain other sodas (check the ingredients list)

Hot dogs

Lentils

Macaroni and cheese

Meats such as ham that are "enhanced" (injected with water and other ingredients)

Milk, cheese, yogurt, and other dairy foods

Nuts and nut butters, including peanut butter

Organ meats, such as liver

Pizza

Processed foods containing preservatives and additives

Sardines

Seeds

Wheat germ

Whole-grain bread

Whole-grain pasta and noodles

LOW-SODIUM FOOD SOURCES

Dishes made with fresh meat and vegetables but no salt, including casseroles, soups, sauces, and salad dressings

Eggs

Fresh beef, fish, pork, and poultry

Fresh fruits and vegetables, including garlic and onion

Lemon juice

Low- or no-sodium seasoning blends

HIGH-SODIUM FOODS TO AVOID

Bouillon cubes

Canned and dehydrated soups, broths, and gravies

Canned vegetables, unless the label specifies "no added salt"

Cheese

Cured and processed meats, such as cold cuts, bacon, and salami, unless the label specifies "no added salt"

Frozen meals

Marmite yeast extract

Pickled foods such as olives and dill pickles

Saltwater crab

Snack foods such as chips and pretzels

Soy sauce and tamari

Table salt

References

American Dietetic Association. "Position of the American Dietetic Association: Vegetarian Diets." *Journal of the American Dietetic Association*. Vol. 109, No. 7 (July 2009): 1266–1282.

Bailey, James L., and Franch, Harold A. "Nutritional Considerations in Kidney Disease: Core Curriculum 2010." *American Journal of Kidney Diseases*. Vol. 55, No. 6 (June 2010): 1146–1161.

Bowman, S., et al. "Fast Food Consumption of U.S. Adults: Impact on Energy and Nutrient Intakes on Overweight Status." *Journal of the American College of Nutrition*. Vol. 23, No. 2 (2004): 163–168.

Brenner, Barry M. "Nutritional Therapy in Renal Disease" (pp. 2298–2327) and "Prescribing Drugs in Renal Disease" (pp. 2606–2642). In *The Kidney*. Sixth Edition. Saunders, 2000.

Brownell, Kelly D., and Koplan, Jeffrey J. "Front of Package Nutrition Labelling—An Abuse of Trust by the Food Industry?" *The New England Journal of Medicine*. Vol. 364, No. 25 (June 23, 2011): 2373–2375.

Clinical Guidelines on the Identification, Evaluation, and Treatment of Overweight and Obesity in Adults—The Evidence Report. National Institutes of Health.

Cohen, Pieter A. "Assessing Supplement Safety—The FDA's Controversial Proposal." *The New England Journal of Medicine*. Vol. 366, No. 25 (February 2, 2012): 389–391.

Dallongeville, J., et al. "Cigarette Smoking Is Associated With Unhealthy Patterns of Nutrient Intake: A Meta-Analysis." *The Journal of Nutrition*. Vol. 128, No. 9 (September 1998): 1450–1457.

Danovitch, Gabriel M. *Handbook of Kidney Transplantation*. Fourth Edition. Lippincott Williams & Wilkins Handbook Series, 2005.

Greenberg, Arthur, Editor. Maroni, Bradley J. "Nutrition and Renal Disease" (pp. 440–447). In *Primer on Kidney Disease*. Second Edition. Academic Press, 1998.

Hakim, Raymond M., and Levin, Nathan. "Malnutrition in Hemodialysis

Patients." *American Journal of Kidney Diseases*. Vol. 21, No. 2 (February 1993): 125–137.

Institute of Medicine, Food and Nutrition Board. *Dietary Reference Intakes for Calcium, Phosphorus, Magnesium, Vitamin D and Fluoride*. Washington, DC: National Academy Press, 1999.

International Bottled Water Association. Bottled Water. www.bottledwater.org

Jalal, D., et al. "Increased Fructose Associates With Elevated Blood Pressure." *Journal of the American Society of Nephrology*. Vol. 21 (2010): 1543–1549.

Johnson, R., et al. "The Effect of Fructose on Renal Biology and Disease." *Journal of the American Society of Nephrology*. Vol. 21, No. 12 (December 2010): 2036–2039.

Katz, David L. *Nutrition in Clinical Practice*. Second Edition. Lippincott Williams and Wilkins, 2008.

Knight, E., et al. "The Impact of Protein Intake on Renal Function Decline in Women with Normal Renal Function for Mild Renal Insufficiency." *Annals of Internal Medicine*. Vol. 138, No. 6 (2003): 460–467.

Ma, J., et al. "Antioxidant Intakes and Smoking Status: Data from the Continuing Survey of Food Intakes by Individuals 1994–1996." *The American Journal of Clinical Nutrition*. Vol. 71, No. 3 (March 2000): 774–780.

Malik, V., et al. "Intake of Sugar-Sweetened Beverages and Weight Gain: A Systematic Review." *The American Journal of Clinical Nutrition*. Vol. 84, No. 2 (August 2006): 274–288.

McCarron, David A., et al., Editors. *Nutrition and Blood Pressure Reviews*. National Kidney Foundation. Vol. 4, No. 3 (Autumn 1994): 1–5.

Mitch, William E., and Ikizler, T. Alp. *Handbook of Nutrition and the Kidney*. Sixth Edition. Lippincott Williams and Wilkins, 2010.

Moe, S.M., et al. "Vegetarian Compared with Meat Dietary Protein Source and Phosphorus Homeostasis in Chronic Kidney Disease." *Clinical Journal of the American Society of Nephrology*. Vol. 6, No. 2 (February 2011): 257–264.

Morbidity and Mortality Weekly Report. Vol. 54, No 37 (Sept 23, 2005).

Morbidity and Mortality Weekly Report. Vol., 57, No. 17 (May 2, 2008).

National Kidney Foundation. *A Guide to GFR Estimates. Chronic Kidney Disease Screening Essentials*.

National Kidney Foundation. KDOQI Clinical Practice Guidelines and Clinical Practice Recommendations for Diabetes and Chronic Kidney Disease: 2007.

National Kidney Foundation. KDOQI Clinical Practice Guidelines for Diabetes and CKD, 2012 Update. *American Journal of Kidney Diseases*. Vol. 60, No. 5 (2012): 850–886.

National Kidney Foundation. KDOQI Guidelines. *American Journal of Kidney Diseases*. Vol. 35, No. 6, Supplement (2000): S 27-S 86.

National Kidney Foundation. KDOQI Nutrition Guidelines in Chronic Renal Failure. *American Journal of Kidney Diseases*. Vol. 35, No. 6: S56-S63.

National Kidney Foundation. *Reducing Mortality and Morbidity in Early Chronic Kidney Disease. Practical Strategies for Primary Care. Clinical Handbook.* 2009.

Pagenkemper, Joni. "Planning a Vegetarian Renal Diet." *Journal of Renal Nutrition*. Vol. 5, No. 4 (October 1995): 234–238.

Report of the DGAC (Dietary Guidelines Advisory Committee) on the Dietary Guidelines for Americans, 2010. www.dietaryguidelines.gov

Rettig, Richard A., et al. *Chronic Kidney Disease—A Quiet Revolution in Nephrology: Six Case Studies.* http://www.rand.org/pubs/technical_reports/TR826.html

Rosen, Clifford J. "Vitamin D Insufficiency." *The New England Journal of Medicine.* Vol. 364, No. 3 (January 2011): 248–254.

The Seventh Report of the Joint National Committee on Prevention, Detection, Evaluation, and Treatment of High Blood Pressure (JNC 7). Bethesda, MD: National Heart, Lung, and Blood Institute, 2003. NIH Publication 03–5233.

Stein, Joel. "Where's the Beet?" *Time.* Aug 23, 2010.

"Strategies to Promote the Availability of Affordable Healthier Food and Beverages." *Morbidity and Mortality Weekly Report.* Vol. 58, No. RR-7 (July 24, 2009): 7–18.

United States Environmental Protection Agency. Ground Water and Drinking Water. http://water.epa.gov/drink/index.cfm

Uribarri, J., et al. "Restriction of Dietary Glycotoxins Reduces Excessive Advanced Glycation End Products in Renal Failure Patients." *Journal of the American Society of Nephrology.* Vol. 14, No. 3 (2003): 728–731.

U.S Department of Health & Human Services. Dietary Guideline for Americans 2005. http://www.health.gov/dietaryguidelines/dga2005/document/

USDA National Nutrient Database for Standard Reference. Last modified Dec 7, 2011. www.nal.usda.gov/fnic/foodcomp/search

Vartanian, L., et al. "Effects of Soft Drink Consumption on Nutrition and Health: A Systematic Review and Meta-Analysis." *American Journal of Public Health.* Vol. 97, No. 4 (April 2007): 667–675.

Warnock, David G., and Drueke, Tilman B. "Introduction to the Third Annual Rostand Vitamin D Symposium." *Clinical Journal of the American Society of Nephrology.* Vol. 5, No. 9 (September 2010): 1696–1722.

Wenzel, Ulrich O., et al. "My Doctor Said I Should Drink a Lot! Recommendations for Fluid Intake in Patients with Chronic Kidney Disease." *Clinical Journal of the American Society of Nephrology.* Vol. 1 (2006): 344–346.

Wojcikowski, K., et al. "Medicinal Herbal Extracts—Renal Friend or Foe?" *Nephrology.* Vol. 9, No. 6 (2004): 313.

Worcester, Elaine M., and Coe, Fredric L. "Calcium Kidney Stones." *The New England Journal of Medicine.* Vol. 363 (2010): 954–963.

Wrone, Elizabeth, and Lentine, Krista. "Nutritional Interventions to Reduce Cardiovascular Risk in Chronic Renal Failure." *Nephrology Rounds.* The Division of Nephrology, Stanford University School of Medicine. Vol. 4, No. 2 (February 2001).

Zeng, D., et al. "Dietary Therapy in Hypertension." *The New England Journal of Medicine.* Vol. 363, No. 16 (2010): 1580–1583.

About the Author

Mandip S. Kang MD, FASN, first became interested in nutrition during medical school, and later gained valuable experience in using kidney diets during his training as a kidney specialist at Wake Forest University School of Medicine. He pursued his passion for teaching and joined the Nephrology Faculty at the University of Utah School of Medicine, where he was a Clinical Assistant Professor. He has served as a Managing Partner at Southwest Kidney Institute in Phoenix, one of the largest nephrology practices in the country, and is a Clinical Assistant Professor at Midwestern University's College of Osteopathic Medicine. Dr. Kang is Board Certified in Internal Medicine and Nephrology, and is also a Fellow of the American Society of Nephrology (FASN). He has been practicing nephrology for over twenty years and was selected Top Doctor in his specialty by *Phoenix* magazine.

The author's lifelong mission is to understand and meet the unique healthcare needs of kidney patients. He works closely with dietitians and enjoys teaching his patients how to manage and slow the progression of kidney disease through nutritional and lifestyle changes. Dr. Kang lives with his family in Glendale, Arizona.

$\mathcal{I}$ndex

SMOOTHIES FOR KIDNEY HEALTH
A Delicious Approach to the Prevention and Management of Kidney Problems and So Much More

Victoria L. Hulett, JD and Jennifer L. Waybright, RN

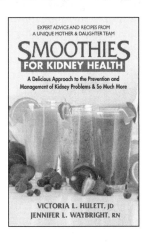

Smoothies for Kidney Health is a very special recipe book. It is expertly put together by a kidney donor who is a registered nurse, and her mom, the recipient of her kidney. Together, they have taken their knowledge and experience to create an information resource and cookbook for all those suffering from chronic kidney disease (CKD).

People who are concerned about kidney health often want to know what they can do to manage their condition and optimize their well-being. *Smoothies for Kidney Health* pairs easy-to-understand dietary information and guidance with luscious kidney-friendly smoothies, helping you gain control over your health deliciously.

$16.95 US • 240 pages • 6 x 9-inch quality paperback • ISBN 978-0-7570-0411-7

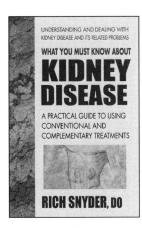

WHAT YOU MUST KNOW ABOUT KIDNEY DISEASE
A Practical Guide to Using Conventional & Complementary Treatments

Rich Snyder, DO

While the news that you or a loved one has kidney disease can be shocking, for over 26 million Americans, it is a reality. After the initial diagnosis and over the years that follow, patients and their families usually have a myriad of questions about treatment options. Written by kidney specialist Dr. Rich Snyder, *What You Must Know About Kidney Disease* is designed not only to answer these questions, but also to provide the up-to-date information you need to cope with this potentially devastating problem.

There is so much you can do to positively affect both your kidney health and your overall well-being. *What You Must Know About Kidney Disease* provides you with the knowledge you need to be a wise participant in your own health care.

$17.95 US • 192 pages • 6 x 9-inch quality paperback • ISBN 978-0-7570-0326-4

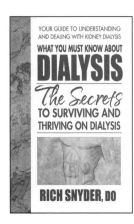

WHAT YOU MUST KNOW ABOUT DIALYSIS
The Secrets to Surviving and Thriving on Dialysis
Rich Snyder, DO

Dialysis is a life-saving technique. If you've been told that you must begin treatment, though, there's probably a good deal you have to learn before you take the next step. *What You Must Know About Dialysis* is designed to provide the up-to-date information you need to understand the process of dialysis, make smart choices, and confidently deal with the many aspects of your treatment plan.

For most people, dialysis is an unplanned and uncharted journey. Whether you are already on dialysis or are just learning about this treatment, *What You Must Know About Dialysis* lights the path ahead by combining rock-solid information with effective strategies that can help you not just survive, but truly thrive on dialysis.

$17.95 US • 208 pages • 6 x 9-inch quality paperback • ISBN 978-0-7570-0349-3

A GUIDE TO COMPLEMENTARY TREATMENTS FOR DIABETES
Using Natural Supplements, Nutrition, and Alternative Therapies to Better Manage Your Diabetes
Gene Bruno, MS, MHS

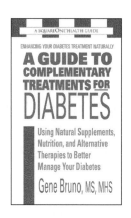

If you are one of the 18 million Americans who have diabetes, you are probably managing your condition with the help of a healthcare professional. But while standard programs can control diabetes, they are not always effective at preventing the serious, life-altering complications that often arise from the disorder—complications such as neuropathies, cardiovascular issues, circulation problems, retinopathy, and weight gain. Fortunately, there are options that can stave off or decrease the severity of diabetes-related problems. In *A Guide to Complementary Treatments for Diabetes,* integrative medical researcher Gene Bruno offers effective, natural ways to complement your current diabetes program and improve your health.

With *A Guide to Complementary Treatments for Diabetes,* you can do more than hope for the best. Now, you can be an active and effective member of your diabetes management team.

$7.95 US • 240 pages • 4 x 7-inch mass paperback • ISBN 978-0-7570-0322-6

GLYCEMIC INDEX FOOD GUIDE
For Weight Loss, Cardiovascular Health, Diabetic Management, and Maximum Energy
Dr. Shari Lieberman

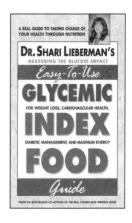

The glycemic index (GI) is an important nutritional tool. By indicating how quickly a given food triggers a rise in blood sugar, the GI enables you to choose foods that can help you manage a variety of conditions and improve your overall health.

Written by a leading nutritionist, this book was designed as an easy-to-use guide to the glycemic index. It first answers commonly asked questions, ensuring that you understand the GI and know how to use it. It then provides both the glycemic index and the glycemic load of hundreds of foods and beverages, including raw foods, cooked foods, and combination foods. Whether you are interested in controlling your glucose levels to manage your diabetes, lose weight, increase heart health, or enhance your well-being, the *Glycemic Index Food Guide* is the best place to start.

$7.95 US • 160 pages • 4 x 7-inch mass paperback • ISBN 978-0-7570-0245-8

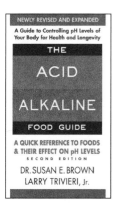

THE ACID-ALKALINE FOOD GUIDE
SECOND EDITION
A Quick Reference to Foods & Their Effect on pH Levels
Susan Brown, PhD, and Larry Trivieri, Jr.

In the last few years, researchers have increasingly reported the importance of acid-alkaline balance. *The Acid-Alkaline Food Guide* was designed as an easy-to-follow guide to the most common foods that influence your body's pH level.

Now in its Second Edition, this bestseller begins by explaining how the acid-alkaline environment of the body is influenced by foods. It then presents a list of thousands of foods and their acid-alkaline effects. Included are not only single foods, such as fruits and vegetables, but also popular combination foods, common fast foods, and even international fare. Updated information also explores (and refutes) the myths about pH balance and diet, and guides you to supplements that can help your body achieve a healthy pH level.

$8.95 US • 224 pages • 4 x 7-inch mass paperback • ISBN 978-0-7570-0393-6